AYURVEDIC AAHAR :
The Scientific Diet

Indian Medical Science Series No.145

AYURVEDIC AAHAR : The Scientific Diet

Prof. Dr. P. H. Kulkarni

Dr. Mahesh Sabade

Dr. Madhura Bhide

Dr. Pradnya Akkolkotkar

Sri Satguru Publications
A Division of
Indian Books Centre
Delhi, India

Published by
Sri Satguru Publications,
Indological and Oriental Publishers
A Division of
Indian Books Centre
40/5, Shakti Nagar,
Delhi-110007
India

Email: ibcindia@vsnl.com
Website: http://www.indianbookscentre.com

First Edition : Pune 2000
Second Edition : Delhi 2002

ISBN 81-7030-739-2

Printed at Chawla Offset Printers, Delhi 110 052

Acknowledgements

A number of individuals and institutions have helped us in carrying out this work successfully. First we must thank our first author Prof. Dr. P.H. Kulkarni in bringing the subject for such an interesting work, followed by our thanks to Mr. Alok kumar Kanungo for his sincere effort, visualization and implementation of the project. The work is financed and sheltered by Ayurveda Research Institute (ARI), Ayurveda Rasashala, and Ayurveda Academy. We are extremely grateful to all these institutions for their valuable and timely support.

We have received assistance from many of our colics in ARI. Among these mention should be made of Dr. B.B. Date for permitting the project to carry put in ARI; Dr. (Mrs.) Pradnya Akkolkotkar for co-ordianting; Dr. Tanuja Nesari & Dr. Sadanand Despande, respective research guides of Dr. Madhura Bhide and Dr. Mahesh sabade; Drs. Yogesh Kale, Manjiri Kulkarni, Ghanashyam Marda, Suraj Marda & Kedar Shende for Research help; Prof. Damle Govind, Mrs. Manjiri Pandharpurkar & Mrs. Kalyani Patne for translation work for the dictionary module. Our grateful thanks are due to all of them.

The people who helped us by encouraging with important suggestion and providing certain rare research material are Drs. Jayant Deopujari, Mandar Akkolkotkar, (Mrs.) Vineeta Bendale, Yogini Patil, and Ajit Kolatkar. We sincerely thank all of them.

We must record our grateful thanks to Mrs. Pushpa Gaikawad for helping in all the way she can; Ms. Shahida Ansari for some important suggestions and photography; Drs. Swati Gadgil & Ashwini Agate for providing some unavailable photos and Ms. Vidyut Kulkarni again for neat photography.

Mrs. Sinnarkar of ARI, Smt. Marathe & Smt. Pawar of Nanal hospital also deserve out thanks for their kind help.

CONTENTS

INTRODUCTION

Introduction to Ayurveda

India, the land of rich culture and heritage has a tradition of a lifestyle and healing science, different from the existing modern medicine - AYURVEDA. It has originated several thousand years ago.

Dharma (to follow the spiritual, social and moral tenets and duties towards the self and others), Artha (to earn livelihood), Kama (all kinds of desires) and Moksna (salvation i.e. to break the cycle of birth, death and rebirth) are the four objectives of human life, which can only be achieved through good health and Ayurveda is the key to good health.

This oldest science of life has originated from the gods. It was initially perceived by Lord Brahma, which he further taught to Daksha Prajapati, who passed on this invaluable knowledge to Ashwinikumar and they taught it to Lord Indra.

The further hierarchy of Ayurvedic intellectuals in different Ayurvedic texts varies. As per Sushrut Samhita, Lord Indra taught it to Lord Dhanvantari. As per Charak Samhita, Bharadwaj (Atreya) learnt it from Lord Indra while Brahmavaivarta-puran considers Ayurveda to be the composition by Bhaskar on the advice of Daksha Prajapati.

Ayurveda understands human physiology in the form of panchamahabhutas (five elements) which are also the basis of mother nature.

Panchamahabhutas which constitute the universe as well as human being are:

Aakash (Ether)
Vayu (Air)
Tej (Fire)
Jala (Water) and
Prithvi (Earth)

These Panchamahabhutas are Omni potent & occur in infinite varieties/ proportions in which each has its own quantities and attributes.

Aakash: In the structure of the Universe aakash represents the space whose essential quality is sound. The characteristics are- light, fine, smooth and soft with effects such as porous, lightness and producing.

Vayu: Vayu represents motion in the universe whose essential quality is touch. This mahabhut represents the principle of propulsion. The main characteristics are- light, colds, dry, rough and fine. The main effects are stimulating motion and activating.

Tej: This mahabhut represents energy in the structure of the universe. The essential quality is Appearance. This represents the principle of conversion and transformation. Hot, sharp, fine, light, dry and clear are the main characteristics of fire. Heats producing and stimulating are the main effects of Tej.

Jala: This mahabhut represents cohesion whose essential quality is taste and is related to the Moon. The main characteristics are liquidity, cold, slow, soft and unctuous. And the main effects of this mahabhut are moistening and dissolving.

Pruthvi: This mahabhut represents Mass and essential quality is smell. It represents the principle of solidity. Heavy, solid, hard, slow, rough and clear are the main characteristics of pruthvi. And growth along with stimulation is the main effects of this mahabhut.

Bodily constituents like doshas, dhatus and malas are the representations of panchamahabhutas.
Doshas viz. vata, pitta and kapha are the biological humours, which perform bodily functions i.e. synthesis of seven dhatus and also malas, the waste products. Doshas alongwith the their subtypes are as follows:

1. Vata: It represents the capacity, which controls all the activities of the body. It is predominant in the region below the umbilicus.

   a. Pran vayu a subtype of vata dosha performs following functions at the site of chest region- respiration, ingestion of food, controlling of sense, memory, intelligence and cardiovascular system, other such as sneezing, swallowing , spitting etc.
   b. Udan vayu also resides within the chest and performs functions from navel to nasal area. The functions include speech, expression, strength, complexion, memory etc.
   c. Saman vayu- This subtype of vata dosha resides in the abdomen. It plays a vital role in the digestion process in accordance with agni (digestive capacity).
   d. Vyan vayu- It resides at the cardiac region and it functions throughout the body. It is responsible for various movements in the body such as yawning, blinking of eyes and circulation of blood.

e. Apan vayu- It functions below the region of umbilicus. The functions are defaecation, micturation, parturation, ejaculation of seminal fluids and menstruation.

2. Pitta: It represents the capacity of conversion through digestion. Pitta lies mainly in the region between umbilicus and heart.

   a. Pachak pitta- It lies between the stomach and umbilicus. It controls preliminary food breakdown and conversion; imparts energy to other subtypes of pitta dosha and regulates the temperature of the body.
   b. Ranjak pitta- It's functional site is said to be in spleen and liver. The red colour of the blood is a physiological effect of Ranjak pitta.
   c. Sadhak pitta- It is located within the vital organs- Heart and brain where it performs the functions of memory, intelligence, art appreciation etc.
   d. Alochak pitta- It is located within the eyes and performs the visual activities.
   e. Bhrajak pitta- This pitta underlies whole skin. It controls temperature and complexion of the skin; important in the absorption of massage oils, balms, ointments and produces skin colour and body aura.

3. Kapha: It represents the capacity to cohesion. In kapha dosha Pruthvi and Jala Mahabhut are predominant. Kapha dosha is primarily located in the thoracic cavity, head and neck.

   a. Avalambak kapha: It lies in the chest region. It controls the secretions which protect the visceral organs from wear and tear. It also helps in the proper functioning of heart.
   b. Kledak kapha: This subtype of kapha dosha is responsible for making food slimy and hence, easy for digestion. This Kledak kapha is situated in the aamashay.
   c. Bodhak kapha: Tongue, which is the site of bodhak kapha, does the function of perception of taste.
   d. Shleshak kapha: It is situated at the site of joints and carries out swift movements by lubrication.
   e. Tarpak kapha: This subtype of kapha dosha mainly nourishes the sense organs and majjadhatu.

Dhatus: These are the constituents of the body that hold the body for the physiological functions. These are well explained physiologically rather than anatomically. Rasa, rakta, mansa, meda, asthi, majja and shukra are the seven dhatus. These have resemblance to and can be taken as plasına, blood tissue, muscle tissue, bone tissue, nervous tissue, reproductive potential of each cell (& semen) respectively.

Mala: These are the waste products excreted after digestion. Purisha (stools), mutra (urine), and sweda (sweat) are the three malas. The commingled state of these constituents with a sound mind makes a perfect human being.

In brief Ayurveda is a science which takes care of the physical and mental wellbeing of an individual. It makes us understand more about ourselves with respect to nature. It will be a very narrow minded view to see Ayurveda, only as a treatment for disease. Metaphysically it covers a very broad aspect. Disease can be thought as a state of body, which a human being transpires to. Ayurveda heals a human being and not only the diseased state.

Introduction to Aahar

The healthy life is primarily dependant on three fundamental activities, which are *Nidra* (sound sleep), *Brahmacharya* (Balanced sexual life), and *Ahar* (Balanced Diet).

The importance of aahar is being underestimated in the fast moving modern world. The customs in eating, the ways of cooking, eating habits of the fast moving modern world are changing for the worse; and so to increase awareness about a balanced and nutritious diet, we are taking a step in that direction.

A good diet is merely combination of foods, which supply the materials vital to the body for its well being. A diet in which various foodstuffs are mixed in suitable proportions to carry out adequately the functions of bodybuilding, energy yielding, and mind nourishing is known as a balanced diet. Good nutrition depends on the capacity for proper digestion and utilisation of food. The presence or absence of a disease, quality of sleep and the mental status of an individual affect this capacity.

Ayurveda primarily aims at the maintenance of health for which it suggests a specific lifestyle. Aahar is the major contributing factor in it. Unlike plants, you cannot utilise the energy of sunlight to provide energy for your own needs. However aahar is the only source of energy for performing the biological work. In Ayurveda good health can be maintained by replenishment of dhatus through proper diet. Ayurveda addresses human body as a complex union of panchamahabhutas. Similarly the universe is also composed of Panchamahabhutas.

Aahar we consume is nothing but the supply of necessary panchamahabhutas. Hence the diet pattern changes from person to person according to his constitution. Intake of aahar depends on agni (digestive capacity). The digestive capacity varies from season to season. This implies that the diet pattern should be changed from season to season. Unlike other pathies mind has an indiscriminate role in maintenance of health according Ayurveda. Ayurveda describes three characteristics of mind viz. satva, raja and tama. The characteristics of mind are enhanced or deleted according to the diet you choose.

Ayurveda has laid simple basic principles related to the properties, preparation and consumption of aahar. Summarising, we can say that agni is a major contributing factor in the consumption of aahar. The aahar consumed ignoring the digestive capacity may lead to various disorders. However a well planned diet helps in restoring the health. Such a planned diet complements to the medicines in the diseased.

Ignorance to the dietary regimen in the modern era has motivated us to concentrate on this subject. This presentation is an unique effort towards creating awareness about aahar, and hence a healthy life.

Ancient Texts

1. Pakadhikaranam
Author - Anonymous

Author begins with salutation to Goddess 'Annapurna' (Goddess of food). He has elaborately explained various 'pakas' - jellies with ash gourd, cumin seeds, etc. He has also explained the dietary regimen as per six seasons.

2. Pakaadhikara
Period 1820-21 AD.

This is a continuation of Pakaadhikaranam with description about more jellies - viz., of coconut, dry ginger, castor etc.

3. Paakadhikara
Period approximately 1746 AD.

Author has explained 46 pakas with their medicinal properties e.g., jelly of dates in anaemia, jelly of garlic in vatavyadhi, etc.

4. Paakavali
Period: 18th century.

Author has described jellies of fruits such as banana, coconut etc. and 'avaleha kalpana'.

5. Pakadhikara from yogaçhintamani compiled by Harsakirti chief of the 'Tapogana' from Nagpur. Collection of pakas already covered in earlier texts.

6. Pakamartanda
Period: 18th century.
Author - Anonymous.

The author has described almost all the pakas known until 18th century. This is one of the most comprehensive works dealing with various Ayurvedic preparations, keeping in view their nutritional value, taste, curative properties and their utility in maintaining sound health.

7. Vividhapakabhasma tailadinirmanam

This text describes the processes of preparations of oils, pakas etc. with the proportions of ingredients used.

8. <u>Bhima bhojana koutuhalam</u>
Author - Vaidyadeshika

This text mainly describes the medicinal recipes; easy ways for the digestion etc. The author has given the ways of mixing different food stuffs so that their combination will help easy digestion.

9. <u>Kshiradi prakaranam</u>
Different varieties of milk of various animals as well as their other products are described in a very systematic manner.

10. <u>Vastugunaaguna</u>
The author has introduced to the basic qualities of the entire range of food stuffs, their nutritive and curative values.

11. <u>Shakaguna</u>
Author - Anonymous
The author has described the qualities of vegetables such as red sorrel, bottle gourd, curry leaves, amaranth etc.

12. <u>Vyanjanvarga</u>
Author - Susena

The author has explained various recipes in it viz., shrikhand, kadhi (buttermilk curry), buttermilk etc.

13. <u>Annapaanvidhi</u>
Author - Susena

The author has described the basic qualities of the different types of food such as milk, water, curds, butter-milk, butter, ghee, oils, wine, sugarcane, grains, vegetables, fruits, pulses, condiments, flesh of many animals etc. Also the eating rituals are described such as betel-chewing after food, having some mouth freshener after food, etc. The author ends the description with some powders (churnas) which are useful for digestion.

14. <u>Kshemakutuhal</u>

The author has explained the allied aspects of cooking and consumption. One can find discussions about the utensils to be used for cooking; the servants qualities who cook the food; various non-veg recipes; medicinal preparations etc.

15. Bhojanakutuhal
Author - Raghunath Ganesh Navahasta or Navathe
Period: 17th century.

This is one of the earliest texts on diet. Author has explained various rituals of food consumption; properties of food grains; various non vegetarian and vegetarian recipes with their properties, etc. The author has also explained the know how about curds and its preparations.

16. Ruchivadhugalaratnamala

This is the most recent text on this subject. The author has covered almost all the topics related to food e.g. about utensils, servants, the medicinal properties of recipes, cooking etc.

17. Takrapanavidhi
Author - Parashar muni

This is the text that is fully devoted to the details about 'Buttermilk'. He has explained the properties of buttermilk prepared from the milk of various animals.

18. Tambulakalpasangrah
Author - Nrusimhabhatta,

This script has detailed description about 'paan'. The benefits, properties, contraindications, timings are explained in it.

19. Tambulmanjiri

This is another text completely devoted to 'paan' or tambul and its medicinal values. The author has given social customs and traditions about 'paan'.

Experts Comments

Prof. Dr. Alaa A. Kaid, Kreuzstrasse 70, 42277 Wupperital, Germany.
Digestion is the most vital process in our body that converts the food into the bodily constituents. Hence aahar should be taken depending upon the digestive capacity. Digestive capacity is a very subjective concept and that is why a diet cannot be the same for everyone.

Angela Sanz, Director, Escuela International De La Ayurvedica, C/Banys 98-08530, La Garriga, Barcelona, Spain.
Relation of mind and diet in various ways is a new concept to the modern world of medicine and Ayurveda has proven it clinically.

Dr. Massimo Moresi, Centro Dl. Ricerca, Europea Dl Ayurveda, V.Delle-Lame 76 INT, 50100 Firenze.
Consumption of ghee in appropriate quantity everyday helps to keep the immunity in good shape. This is an accepted fact that cow's ghee contains 'Omega-3', which does not create harmful cholesterol (LDL).

Lucia Tomasini, Cilus Saqnvito Di Narni, 50535 (IERNI), Italy.
It is a myth that Ayurveda emphasises only on vegetarianism. However it advocates non-vegetarian food at many places. The diet should be chosen as per the digestive capacity, the place, weather, disease if any etc.

Shanti Govans, The Meditation Institute, Po. Box. 3512, Southport, Queensland 4215, Australia.
Medicines and diet go hand in hand in treatment of any diseases. So proper dietetic regimen should be followed correctly for the faster results.

B. R. Lalitha, No 4 Chickanna Cottages, Loop lane off Racecourse Road, Bangalore – 560009, India.
The nature of food preparation is very important because body is resultant of Aahara. Aahara is nourishing, energy gaining, replenishing; it sustains the body, increases the memory, enhances the life span, increases agni, brings complexion to skin, and increases the mental faculty.

Dr. Deopujari Jayant, Igg, Shankar Nagar, Nagpur, India.
The post Panchakarma dietary regimen is called as sansarjan kram. During vaman and virechan karma there is much stress on Annavaha srotas and the digestive fire gets slowed. Hence it is advised to follow the dietetic regimen with *peya, vilepi* etc. in three, two or one mealtime respectively according to the degree of evacuation like superior, medium or inferior.

Dr. B.K. Bhagwat
The types of food items that can cause cancer is unanswearable. But non-vegeterian diet, too much spicy substances and non-residue diets after prolonged administration may cause cancer. Tobacco and cigaratte ,definitely cause cancer of mouth and the oesophagus and respiratory tract.

Dr. M.B. Akkalkotkar, Ayurveda Rasashala, 25 Karve Road, Pune, India
There are various vegetables explained in charak samhita, which are difficult to find. We all should take a step towards cultivation of such herbs all over the world.

Farida Irani, 80 Coonara Avenue, West Pannant Hills, NSW. 2125, Australia.
Water is a very essential nutrient for our body and any soft drink or beer cannot replace it. Water should be consumed at least during the meals. I also recomendd some aromatic oils which are beneficial in internal oleation of the body and cleaning as well.

Dr. Khasgiwale Dhananjay, 570 NarayanPeth, Pune – 30, India.
Cooked food is more easily digested and assimilated than raw food. The food processed by heat becomes *laghu* i.e., lighter to digest. Especially meat items should be cooked properly before consumption.

Dr Scott Gerson, Ayurvedic Medicineo of NewYork, Suite – 1, 13 West 9th Street, New York, NY 10011, U.S.A.
Dietetics is an important aspect of Ayurveda as it fulfils the Ayurveda's aim of maintenance of health and treatment of a disease completely.

Dr. Pratichi Sinha, Prachi Inc, The Holistic Rejuvenation Centre, 4898 El Camino Real, Suite – 203, Los Altos, CA 94022, U.S.A.
'Viruddha-aahar' (unhealthy combinations of food) is a unique concept in Ayurveda, which is being overlooked by the modern world of fast food.

Dr. Athique MM, 20 Annes Grove, Great Linford, Milton Keynes MK 14 5DR, London.
Dietetics is being studied from various aspects, but the way Ayurveda understands it is fabulous. Dietetic in Ayurveda can be a complete science in itself.

Gino Veronesi, Ambrosia S.A.S., Prodotti Ayurvedic 1, Via Ricasoli 55, 50122 Firenze, Italy.
India is a land of a number of recipes. Most of them are designed and prepared by keeping the principles of Ayurveda in mind.

Anna Belgium
Everybody should select such a diet, which will be useful for the maintenance of health and prevention of the disease.

Dr. Govind Dandekar
One should see that half of the stomach should be filled with solid or semisolid food, one fourth should be filled with water and remaining quarter portion should be kept empty for air. This will prevent indigestion.

Dr. Rani Pargaokar, Rani Holistic Health Centers, 608 West 81 St. Ave., Merrillville, IN4 6410, U.S.A.
Human being cannot create food for his own use like plants. So he has to take vegetarian or non-vegetarian food items so that he can get raw or basic material, from which he can create substances, which are very much useful for his existence and maintenance.

Anna Salema
The surrounding and atmosphere in the dining room should be clean, cheerful and fragrant.

Dr. S.N. Bhide, 6/63, Tulshibagwale Colony, Hemanti Apartment, Sahakar Nagar 2, Pune - 9.
With the help of horoscope ideal diet can be suggested. This gives information about his/ her srotasa and organs. For an example, Plannetory periods (*Mahadosha*) – there are elevation in *tridosha* as per his/ her period. Accordingly diet can be selected e.g. vata dosha elevation in satrun/ shani period.

Dr. Maneesh Patwardhan, B-3 Prajakta Appartment, Near Vitthal Mandir, Karve Nagar, Pune – 411052.
Administration of IV fluids when agni (digestive fire) is low may be an overload of Aap mahabhuta to the body. Such a condition may cause various disorders like diarrhoea.

Kshitija Bhide, U.S.A.
Don't eat food in hurry or when you are having disturbed state of mind full of tension, stress and emotional outbreaks. Regain peace of mind and then enjoy food with happy mood.

Dr. Suhas Kshirsagar
According to Ayurveda well balanced diet consists of foodstuffs having all the six tastes.

Dr. Vasant Lad, The Ayurveda Institute, Po. Box. 32445, Albu Quer Que, N.M. 87192-1445, USA.
The consumption of aahar is nothing but the supply of panchamahabhutas to the body. The diet should be planned in such a way that the requirement of the body for a particular mahabhuta gets fulfilled.

Ganoo Avinash & Swati
One should not eat the food in hurry or very slowly. Food should be chewed properly.
Christine Reid, Po. Box. 810, 10 Isobel Street, Salisbury S. A. 5108, Australia.
While consuming food the sequence of taking different tastes should be in order of sweet, sour, salty, and pungent, bitter, astringent.

Jennie Trampeva-Radin, Optimum Health Ayurveda Pvt. Ltd., Po. Box. 134, Runple-Mall 5000, S. Australia.
Food should be freshly prepared and served warm. It should contain all the six tastes in proper proportion. Warm food is tasty and intensifies agni, which in turn promotes digestion.

Juliette Parkin, 36 Swiet Ave, Dulwich, South Australia 5065.
Water should be consumed only when you are thirsty. Hot and cold drinks should not be consumed simultaneously.

Emelia Lopresto, 19 Malcolm St., Adilade, Feryden Park, S. Australia.
It is recommended not to sleep within two hours of consumption of food. Daytime sleep is not recommended at all except in summer. In summer also sleep just after lunch is contraindicated.

Rosemarie Urban, 4. Dudley Ave, Prospect 5087, S. Australia.
Consumption of ghee helps the growth of the foetus and hence regular intake in pregnancy is recommended.

Philippe Payet, 233 Rue du Faubourv, Saint Martin, 75010 Paris, France.
It has been mentioned in Ayurveda that if a person suffering from any disease follows strictly the regulation of diet, he may not require any medicine, but if he does not follow the regulation of diet the medicine will be fruitless.

Dr. EBS Premdani, Rijksstraatinieg. 195, 3956 Cm. Leersum, Holland.
After taking food in correct doses a person does not feel sleepy, instead he can easily engage himself in his usual activities.

Dr. Kenneth G. Zysk, Asien Institute, University of Copenhagen, Reifsgade 33. SDK 2300, Kobenhayn, Denmark.

Some food items prepared by mixing two substances in equal amount are contraindicated e.g., honey and ghee. Also diet taken in excess or in fewer amounts than the normal requirement are contraindicated.

Dr. Shubhada Bopegamage, 8331 Brati, SLAVA, Slovaka.
According to Indian customs and tradition, food should be consumed by sitting in '*sukhasan*' i.e. with legs folded below the laps. This helps in digestion of the food.

Swami Jyotirmayanand, Joytinat Centre, Via Balbi 33/29, 16/26 Genova, GE, Italy.
Food is god's own reflection. Let us not waste it and insult it.

Dr. B.B. Date, President ARI, 25 Karve Road, Pune, India.
The amount of food, which without disturbing the equilibrium of dhatus and doshas of the body, gets digested in a proper period of time can be refered to as proper quantity.

W.W. Wicker, Buro Wicker, Nikolaweg – 1, 64287 Darmstadt, Germany.
Aahar is one of the three fundamentals of a healthy life (*Upastambha)* and hence proper dietetic regimen is a pathway towards healthy life.

Dr. Yogesh Kale, ARI, 25 Karve Road, Pune, India
Regular exercise helps to improve the appetite and digestion.

Dr. Ghanashyam Marda, ARI, 25 Karve Road, Pune, India
By following principles of Ayurveda and using some of the spices, all the food items can be made delicious as well as nutritious.

Dr. Pradnya M. Akkalkotkar, Asst. Director, ARI, 25 Karve Road, Pune, India
Newborn babies are totally dependent on the breast milk, and hence during lactation, the dietetic regimen of the mothers should be in such a way that the milk is formed in sufficient quantity and the doshas are well in balance.

Dr. Sadanand Deshpande, HOD, Tilak Ayurveda College, Pune, India.
The dietetic regimen to be followed after Panchakarma procedure has a major role of increasing agni and alleviation of remaining vitiated doshas.

Tami Poran
We have a saying in Herbrew, which means – "It is better to eat less and be satisfied. It is a pity that eating more can cause toxins which are difficult to get rid of………….".

Dr. Magon
The diet pattern should change from season to season as well as place to place, as the strength of agni is variable.

AAHAR AND YOU

Constitution

Prakruti or the constitution is the nature of an individual, which remains unchanged throughout the life. Ayurveda has an individualistic approach to consider each human separately. The doshas dominant at the time of conception determines the prakruti (constitution) of an individual. The other factors responsible for the constitution are:

1. The quality of sperm cell and ovum.
2. The condition of uterus at the time of conception.
3. The dietetic and behavioural pattern of the mother during pregnancy.
4. Influence of panchamahabhutas.

The prakruti thus formed is of seven types depending on the permutations and combinations of doshas. The nomenclature of constitution is done on the basis of dominance of dosha e.g. in vata prakruti vata dosha is dominant. Apart from the doshic prakruti, Ayurveda describes maanas prakruti (constitution of the psyche) also. Satva, Raja and Tama are the three basic constitutions, which are responsible for all the mental activities. Satva is aakash (eather) mahabhut dominant constituent of the mind. When this constituent is dominant in a prakruti, it is termed as 'Satvik prakruti'. The characteristics of this prakruti are as follows:

1. Pure and pious thinking.
2. Theism
3. Studious
4. Reverence for Guru (teacher).
5. Courageous
6. Scientific and rational outlook
7. Tolerant
8. Sweet tongued
9. Liking towards fragrance and flowers
10. Strong memory, intellectual
11. Control over anger, hatred, greed, fear etc.
12. Various forms of bhakti (devotion)
13. Knowledgeable
14. Followers of ideal dietary regimen etc.

Raja guna is vayu and tej mahabhut (air & fire) dominant constituent of the mind. When in a prakruti rajaguna is dominant, it is termed as 'Rajas prakruti'. The characteristics found in this prakruti are as follows:

1. Materialistic desires
2. Short tempered
3. Unpredictable diet intake, liking of pungent taste.
4. Aggressive, hasty
5. Excessive indulgence in sex.
6. Jealousy
7. Adventurous
8. Shameless
9. Lusty etc.

Tama guna is pruthvi mahabhut (earth) dominant constituent of the mind. The prakruti in which tama guna is dominant, is termed as 'Tamas prakruti'. The characteristics of this prakruti are as follows:

1. Lethargy
2. Excessive sleep
3. Idiotic behaviour
4. Coward
5. Inertia
6. Excessive eating
7. Unbalanced
8. Excessive indulgence in sex
9. Atheism etc.

This description gives a brief idea to discover your physical and mental constitution, which will guide you to choose your dietary pattern.

Constitution and Aahar

Aahar is a major contributing factor in the constitution of an individual. Aahar replenishes all the seven dhatus in the body through digestion. A good nutritious aahar is responsible for proper nourishment of the dhatus. Shukra dhatu (reproductive potential) is responsible for fertilisation. Properly nourished shukra dhatu results in a healthy constitution of the offspring.

Doshas, panchamahabhutas as well as mind have influence on the constitution. Aahar keeps these bodily constituents in a state of equilibrium. Thus a healthy body, mind and soul makes a healthy constitution of the offspring. Ayurveda recommends a general dietary regimen according to the constitution. The diet patterns described below are the guidelines to choose your diet according to your constitution. The food stuffs which are not to be consumed in excess are described in don'ts.

Vata

Subject	Don'ts	Do's
Fruits	Most dried fruits, apples, dates-dry, dry figs, pears, watermelon in excess.	Apricot, avocado, banana, berries, Cherrie, coconut, figs, grape fruit, grapes, lemon, mango, sweet melon, oranges, papaya, peaches, pineapple, plums
Vegetables	Raw, frozen, dried veggies, raw cabbage, broccoli, cauliflower, eggplant, lettuce, mushrooms, onions, peppers, potatoes, spinach, tomatoes, sprouts, turnips.	Asparagus, broccoli, beet root, carrot, cucumber, garlic, green beans, leeks, onions, potatoes (sweet), peas, radish, pumpkin.
Legumes	No legumes except lentils (red, black), tofu.	Lentils (red, black), mung beans, tofu
Dairy foods	Hard cheese, powdered milk.	Ghee, buttermilk, and all other foods.
Animal foods	Lamb, rabbit, flesh of the animals which are hyperactive	Beef, chicken, duck, eggs, seafood, turkey
Grains	Barley, corn, millets	Cooked oats, rice, wheat
Nuts	None should be eaten in excess	All in moderate quantity
Spices & condiments	Chocolate, horse radish, chilli, peppers	All spices can be consumed in moderate quantity
Oils		All oils can be consumed.

Kapha

Subject	Don'ts	Do's
Fruits	Banana, coconut, figs, kiwifruit, oranges, papaya, plums, rhubarb, watermelon, custard-apple, pineapple.	Astringent fruits such as apples, berries, cherries, figs-dry, peaches, pears, prunes, raisins.
Vegetables	Cucumber, olives, sweet potatoes, pumpkin, tomatoes, zucchini.	Asparagus, cabbage, eggplant, garlic, mushrooms, potatoes, radishes, spinach, turnip, broccoli, beet root.
Legumes	Kidney beans, soya beans, black lentils.	All can be consumed.
Dairy foods	Curds, hard cheese, mayonnaise, buffalo's milk.	Buttermilk, goat's milk, cow's milk.
Animal foods	Beef, duck, lamb, pork, seafood, flesh of aquatic animals.	Chicken, eggs, rabbit, shrimp.
Grains	Oats - cooked, rice.	Barley, corn, wheat, millets, oats, ragi.
Nuts	No nuts should be consumed	
Spices and condiments	Chocolate, salt, vinegar.	All spices can be consumed.
Oils	Coconut oil, castor oil.	Almond, corn, sunflower, sesame oil, mustard oil, safflower.

Pitta

Subject	Don'ts	Do's
Fruits	Sour fruits such as apricots, berries, banana, cherries, grape fruit, lemons, oranges, peaches, plums, pineapples, cranberries.	Apples, berries, apricots, coconut, mango, pears, raisins, prunes, watermelon, pomegranate.
Vegetables	Beet roots, carrots, eggplant, garlic, green chillies, olives, raw onions, horse radish, pungent veggies, peppers, radishes, spinach, tomatoes, turnips.	Asparagus, beet root, leafy greens, lettuce, mushrooms, onions, potatoes, pumpkin, sprouts, broccoli, artichokes, zucchini.
Legumes	Lentils, miso, soya sauce, soya sausages.	All except lentils.

Dairy foods	Salted butter, curds, cheese, cold milk, sour cream.	Buttermilk, butter without salt, cheese, milk, ghee.
Animal foods	Beef, duck, eggs (yolk), lamb, pork, seafood.	Chickens, eggs, fish, rabbit. Shrimp, turkey.
Grains	Corn, millet, oats, sago, rice.	Barley, rice, wheat, ragi.
Nuts	No nuts should be consumed.	Coconut.
Spices and condiments	No spices.	Coriander, cinnamon, cardamom, fennel can be consumed.
Oils	Sesame, almond, corn, safflower, mustard.	Coconut, olive, sunflower.

Season and Aahar

The dietetic regimen, which we follow in day to day routine, has various effects on our body. The well being of human body is directly dependent upon the type of food we have. Ayurveda suggests some changes in diet one has to make with respect to the season and has detailed scientific description regarding it.

According to the texts, a year comprises of twelve months which are divided into six seasons viz.:- Shishir (Late winter), Vasant (Spring), Greeshma (summer), Varsha (Monsoon/ fall), Sharad (Autumn) and Hemant (Early winter). These seasons are due to the apparent movements of the sun.

'Uttarayan' is a phenomenon where there is an apparent movement of the sun towards Northern Hemisphere. And 'Dakshinayan' is a phenomenon where there is an apparent movement of the sun towards Southern Hemisphere. Uttarayan is the period in which tej and vayu mahabhut are dominant. The dryness of these mahabhutas depletes the unctuousness of the body in turn reducing the strength. Shishir (Late winter), Vasant (Spring), and Greeshma (Summer) are included in this period and the level of dryness increases in the same order.

Dakshinayan is the period in which jala and pruthvi mahabhut are dominant. These mahabhutas enhance the unctuousness thus giving strength to the body. The first season of Dakshinayan is Varsha (monsoon). The cooling properties of rainwater pacify the heat generated in 'Uttarayan' in turn increasing the unctuousness. Varsha (monsoon), Sharad (autumn) and Hemant (early winter) are included in this period. Ayurveda recommends a specific dietary regimen for each season.

The dietary regimen depends upon various factors such as agni, age, strength, constitution desh and season. When an individual is suffering from any ailment, the dietary pattern can be altered to some extent considering the above factors.

Dietetic regimen in Shishir (late winter)

Do's	Don'ts
Unctuous, fresh and warm food.	Cold food stuffs and beverages.
Sweet, sour and salty food can be consumed.	Pungent, bitter and astringent food in excess.
Heavy food such as flesh of lamb, pork, etc. can be consumed.	Dry, light, fermented and stale food.
Fish from lakes being sweet, unctuous and nutritious can be consumed.	Flesh of animals from jangal region e.g. flesh of deer.

Dietetic regimen in Vasant (spring)

Do's	Don'ts
Food prepared from barley and wheat.	Heavy, unctuous and cold food.
Consumption of 'sidhu' (wine prepared from sugarcane).	Food with sweet and sour tastes.
Flesh of birds can be consumed.	Flesh of aquatic animals.
Flesh from rivers being hot and nutritious can be consumed.	

Dietetic regimen in Greeshma (summer)

Do's	Don'ts
Cold and unctuous food should be consumed e.g. cow's ghee, milk etc.	Alcohol should not be consumed.
More liquids should be consumed e.g. Buttermilk.	Salty, sour and pungent food likes ginger.
Mangoes and pomegranate can be consumed.	Spicy, dry, hot and fermented food.
Sweet food stuffs in accordance with agni e.g. sharkarodak.	Flesh of lamb, beef and pork.
Flesh of animals from jangal desh e.g. chicken.	
Fish from ponds being unctuous, sweet and cold can be consumed.	

Dietetic regimen in Varsha (Monsoon)

Do's	Don'ts
Honey should be included in daily diet.	Dry, cold, heavy, food in excess e.g. cheese, curds.
Barley and wheat can be consumed.	Bengal gram, field pea, etc. in excess.
Flesh of animals of jangal desha.	Fermented and stale food.
Pre heated water should be consumed.	Cold beverages in excess.
Milk, ghee, plain butter can be consumed.	
Fish from lakes being aphrodisiac and unctuous can be consumed.	

Dietetic regimen in Sharad (autumn)

Do's	Don'ts
Food stuffs with attributes like sweet, slight bitter, light and cold can be consumed.	Curds, fermented food are strongly contraindicated.
The diet should be consumed in accordance with digestive capacity i.e., in proper proportion.	Food of alkaline nature should not be consumed in excess e.g. radish, salts, drumstick, ginger etc.
Flesh of rabbit, fish of spring water being nutritious for mind and body can be consumed.	Tomato, brinjals. Ladies finger, chillies etc.
Barley, ragi and wheat can be consumed.	Beverages containing sour fruits.
Unctuousness of the flesh of animals of aanup desh.	
Oils can be consumed.	

Dietetic regimen in Hemant (early winter)

Do's	Don'ts
Unctuous, sour and salty food can be consumed.	Dry, cold, light, food in excess.
Flesh of the animals in aanup desh and fish found in wells as they increase kapha and shukra.	Food stuffs with tastes pungent, bitter and astringent in excess.
Various preparations of sugarcane, meat soup, new crops, milk products etc. can be consumed.	Daytime sleep is strongly contraindicated in all seasons except Greeshma (summer), especially after meals.
Lukewarm water should be consumed.	
As the digestive capacity is good, alcohol can be consumed.	

Mind and Aahar

Ayurveda understands mind alongwith the soul as an inseparable characteristic of a live human being. Ayurvedic texts have substantial references to the role of diet in the physical, mental and spiritual wellbeing of an individual. Bhagwad Geeta an ancient scripture states that food affects senses and categorises diet as satvik, rajas and tamas in descending order of its merit.

Mind with the help of aatman (soul) and indriya (sensory and motor organs) perceive the knowledge (sense). The sensory organs are:

1. Ghranendriya (sensory organ of smell)
2. Shrotrendriya (sensory organ of hearing)
3. Sparshanendriya (sensory organ of touch)
4. Chakshurendriya (sensory organ of vision)
5. Rasanendriya (sensory organ of taste).

The motor organs are:

1. Vagendriya	Tongue
2. Paani	Hands
3. Paad	Legs
4. Paayu	Arms
5. Upastha	Penis

Mind is the indriya (organ) which acts both as sensory and motor. It controls various desires i.e., whether to accept or reject a particular thing and to differentiate between. This controlling is termed as 'chintya' which is a subject of mind. This process of acceptance and rejection traverses through following steps:

1. Chintya: Contemplation or planning of a subject.
2. Vicharya: Thinking about the subject.
3. Uhya: Full consideration of the subject.
4. Dheyeya: Considering of the subject as a goal.
5. Sankalpya: Final decisions whether to accept or reject.

This process of decision making is very fast to differentiate. The things favourable to health (mental and physical) should be accepted and thought of. Similarly the things which are not favourable, but accepted and thought of disturb the mental health and subsequently the physical health.

Excessive thinking, lack of thinking, and horrifying thoughts lead to mental stress and other psychological disorders. Ayurveda recommends a behavioural regimen by which mental health can be attained.

Gods, guru (teachers), seers and aged should be worshipped and given due respect. Fire being the symbol of the digestive capacity in the human body should be worshipped. Personal hygiene should be maintained. The guests should be treated with hospitality. He should keep himself away from jealousy, hatred, anger, fears etc. Similarly Ayurveda also recommends dietetic regimen which helps to maintain the mental health.

Hands should be washed upto the elbows, prior to meals. Server and the cook should be mentally sound. The surroundings should be pleasant so as to enhance the digestion. The utensils used for cooking and eating should be clean as regular intake of unclean and untidy food and way of eating may lead to insanity. Stale food, tinned food, preserved food should be avoided as far as possible. Without feeling of hunger, food should not be consumed; especially curds, honey, salt and ghee. Intake of curds is not recommended at night.

Overlooking the above dietetic and behavioural regimen may vitiate the health.

Satva, raja and tama are three attributes of mind. Satva expresses essence, understanding, purity, clarity, compassion and love. Raja implies movement, aggressiveness. And tama manifests ignorance and stabilises the mind. Raja and tama are negative attributes, which destabilise and weaken the mind. Thus satva balances raja as well as tama, and in turn the mind. Ayurveda recommends a specific dietary regimen that will help to enhance the satva attribute of the mind.

Consumption of wheat, barley, rice grains (especially the variety which is harvested in spring), radish, white-goosefoot (Chenopodium album), haritak (Terminalia chebula), amalaki (Emblica officinale), grape raisins, green gram, sugar, cow's milk, butter and ghee; honey, pomegranate, rock salt, various fruit juices etc. Similarly foodstuffs having attributes such as unctuous, sweet taste, light, freshly prepared, easily digestible and vegetarian should be consumed.

Some foodstuffs that aggravate raja attribute are as follows:
Spicy, hot, pungent, salty, kshar (strongly alkaline in nature), onion, garlic, fermented, improperly cooked, over-ripen radish, dry pork, flesh, pepper powder in excess, fish, alcohol prepared from barley, stale food etc. Similarly consumption of food when one is angry, jealous, anxious, sad etc. aggravates raja.

The foodstuffs that aggravate tama attribute are as follows:

Hard cheese, flesh and milk of buffalo, curds, excessive intake of sweet taste, red meat, opium seeds, excessive intake of alcohol, newly harvested grains, flesh of aquatic animals, black gram, jaggery etc.

The foodstuffs with dominance of pruthvi (earth) mahabhut aggravate tama. Ayurveda strongly contraindicates the foodstuffs having attributes such as heavy, dry, rough in excess.

From the above description we come to a conclusion that quality of mind is affected very greatly by the nature of the food we eat. Summarising we can list some of the food stuffs which maintain the health of the psyche.

Do's	Don'ts
Mint, barley, wheat, rice (all grains should be roasted before cooking), plain butter, buttermilk, green gram, drumstick leaves, salads, bottle gourd, snake gourd, bitter gourd, sweet potato, yam, french beans, ginger, fresh turmeric, garlic and basil.	Curds, cabbage, brinjal, vegetables with too many seeds, tea, coffee, cold drinks, ice chilled water, banana with milk, sugarcane juice, fried savories, and snakes, fermented foods, bread, cakes, biscuits, pickles, watermelons, crisples etc.

PRINCIPLES OF AAHAR

Agni

Transformation of Panchabhautic elements in form of food to the panchabhautic elements of the body is known as pachan (digestion). This process of transformation is performed by Agni (the strength by which food nourishes the tissue elements of the body is agni.). Agni which literally means fire, is the digestive capacity in our body, which is also called as jatharagni.

Similarly seven dhatus and five mahabhutas posses digestive capacity for the regeneration of respective dhatu and mahabhutas. Health of an individual is dependent on the proper functioning of the Agni. Sama agni (balanced) helps to maintain the longevity of life and nourish dosha, dhatu and malas.

At the site of umbilicus there are two imaginary concentric circles. The outer one is governed by soma (moon) and the inner one is governed by surya (sun). The agni is situated inside the circle of surya which performs the functions of digestion. The same can be represented automatically in the *grahani.*

Grahani is that part of the intestine which holds the food for digestion. The proper functioning of agni is controlled by three doshas. Pran, apan and saman the subtypes of vata dosha help in improving and maintaining the quality of agni. In the same manner agni performs its functions through pachak pitta a subtype of pitta dosha. Similarly bodhak kapha - a subtype of kapha dosha understands taste of the food which inturn stimulates the agni.

Another subtype of kapha dosha - kledak kapha assists agni in its function by formation of proper bolus of the ingested food.

The maximum time limit for digestion in a healthy individual is four 'yaam' i.e., approximately 12 hours. Physiologically the agni is of four types viz., sama, visham, mand and teekshna. The agni which digests the proper (heavy) as well as improper (light) food in a stipulated time period is sama. The one which is uncertain is the visham agni. It may digest heavy food quickly and light lately.

Manda type of agni is the one which takes a little more time to digest both the qualities of food. Teekshna agni digests both qualities of food in a short period of time. There are many references one can find in Ayurvedic texts about the correlation of agni and disease with respect to an individual.

Basic Principles of Aahar

We get references from Ayurvedic texts in which ancient seers have done a detailed study of basic principles of aahar. The basic principles include the study of the digestive capacity of an individual; rasa (tastes) and other properties of food material which are explained here. Agni is the digestive capacity which converts the food material into a form which is easier to be assimilated and absorbed in the body.

There are six different tastes viz. Madhur (sweet), Amla (sour), Lavan (salty), Katu (pungent), Tikta (Bitter), and Kashay (astringent). Ayurveda advises to have a regular intake of all the six tastes in the dietary pattern. Each rasa is a composite of panchamahabhutas with the dominance of two mahabhutas as stated.

Madhur	Pruthvi (earth) & Jala (water)
Amla	Pruthvi (earth) & Tej (fire)
Lavan	Tej (fire) & Jala (water)
Tikta	Aakash (ether) & Vayu (air)
Katu	Tej (fire) & Vayu (air)
Kashay	Pruthvi (earth) & Vayu (air)

Actions of tastes on the body:

a. Madhur (sweet): It is the taste habitual right from the childhood as it replenishes the dhatus e.g., milk.

b. Amla (sour): Food, which tastes amla, acts as a good appetiser. Most of the herbs, which are sour in taste, are cardiotonics e.g., Amalaki (Emblica officinale).

c. Lavan (salty) - This relishes the food and increases the digestive capacity. It's overuse leads to greying of hair and baldness e.g., common salt.

d. Tikta (bitter) - Though an impleasant taste it rectifies the functions of tongue (perception of taste). Due to excessive intake of tikta rasa, it has negative effects on the body causing depletion of dhatus and various vata disorders e.g. vacha (Acorus calamus).

e. Katu (Pungent) - Intake of this taste elevates the digestive capacity of an individual. This taste makes the food palatable and being dry in nature reduces unctuousness of the body. Overuse of this taste may create depletion of shukradhatu e.g., red chillies.

f. Kashay (astringent) - This taste being dry and cool in nature, has got the property of reducing the flow by constriction. It's overuse causes constipation, excessive thirst, spasmodic pain and angina e.g., betel-nut.

Though Ayurveda recommends the intake of food having all the six tastes, it also recommends that overuse of a single taste should be avoided. The other properties of food material include veery (potency) and vipak (post digestive effect). Indian philosophy understands two vital energies in the universe - solar and lunar. Ayurveda in terms of veerya-ushna (hot) and sheeta (cold) state the same principle. This is the potency of the food or herb by which it acts on the body.

We are aware that the ingested food is acted upon by 'agni' and gets digested, which is assimilated in the body. The concept of vipak can be said as the taste (rasa) attained by the digested food material in the alimentary canal. Though the vipak can not be practically perceived, it can be felt from the effects it has or does on the body. The vipak can either be madhur (sweet), amla (sour) or katu (pungent).

Maintenance of health and treatment of a disease are based on a primordial principle – "samanya vishesh siddhant". This principle states that food with the dominance of a particular mahabhut increases bodily constituent of the same mahabhut quantitatively or qualitatively. Similarly the food with dominance of a particular mahabhut decreases bodily constituent of the opposite mahabhut quantitatively or qualitatively e.g., consumption of meat or black gram increases muscle tissue in the body. And hot milk alleviates vata dosha.

Regarding the preparation of food, Ayurveda has laid some basic rules.

1. Prakruti: This is the nature of the food e.g., black gram by its nature is heavy to digest and hence those having less digestive capacity should not take it.
2. Karana: The process by which the properties of the food material are changed or enhanced are termed as karana. These include washing, cooking, blending, grinding, roasting etc.
3. Sanyog: Sanyog is to combine two different food materials together, e.g., while preparing buttermilk water is added to curds.
4. Rashi: Literal meaning of rashi is quantity. It is taken as the total quantity or the proportion of the ingredients mixed together. The total quantity of food depends upon the digestive capacity of an individual, whereas the proportion of ingredients is usually fixed e.g., in buttermilk one part of curds and four parts of water are taken.
5. Desh: The meaning of the word 'desh' is place. It is taken as the place of the food from where it is originated and the place of consumption. There are three types of desh viz. Aanup, jangal, Sadharan.
   Aanup desh has the dominance of pruthvi and jala mahabhut, hence it is recommended to have hot and unctuous food. Jangal desh has the dominance of tej, aakash and vayu mahabhut, hence cold and unctuous foods are recommended. Sadharan desh has all the mahabhutas in a balanced state.
6. Kaal: Kaal, which literally means time can be taken as seasonal, and the state of the disease. Ayurveda recommends a specific dietary regimen for diurnal, nocturnal, seasonal along with acute and chronic conditions of the disease e.g., consumption of curds, heavy food should be avoided at night.

7. Upayogasanstha: These are the rules for consumption of food. One of the main principles is that the second meal should be taken only after the first has been digested.
8. Upayokta: Upayokta is the person who is going to be benefited by following the rules explained above.

Consumption of Food

Food is classified in three types viz. jaangam, audbhid and parthiv.

Jaangam: The main sources of this type of food are animals, fish, birds, insects etc. e.g., milk, curds, butter, yoghurt, cheese, eggs, honey, flesh etc.

Audbhid: Cereals and pulses are included in this category e.g., wheat, rice grain etc.

Parthiv: Minerals, metals etc. are included in this category e.g., common salt.

According to the effects of the substances shown on the body, food is classified into following types:

1. Shaman: This category includes the food materials, which have suppressant action over the elevated doshas.
2. Kopan: This category includes the food materials, which increase doshas above their normal level.
3. Swasthahita: This category includes those food materials which neither increase nor suppress the level of doshas and thus maintain the balanced state of the body. Similarly aahar can be classified into Hitakara & Ahitakara. The aahar beneficial to an individual according to his constitution is called 'Hitakara aahar'. And the aahar, which is harmful to an individual according to his constitution, is called 'Ahitakara aahar'.

Apart from the properties of food, Ayurveda also explains various aspects in eating, cooking etc. Freshly prepared warm food is advised as it increases the digestive capacity, alleviates vata and kapha dosha.

Unctuous food is a good appetiser, it increases strength and improves complexion. Depending upon the digestive capacity, the quantity of food should be decided. Such a well proportionate food helps in proper digestion by maintaining the strength agni. Most of the diseases are the progeny of improper functioning of agni. Ayurveda specifically elaborates the signs of completion of digestion which are belching without any taste or odour; feeling of lightness in the abdomen as well as in the body and feeling of hunger. The next meal should not be consumed before observing these signs.

The ingredients in the recipes should not be of opposite veerya (potency i.e., hot and cold). If done so it is nothing but 'viruddha - aahar' (wrong combined food). Proper digestion also depends upon well equipped place and the place favourable for your mental conditions.

Hurriedly eating is strenuous for the digestive capacity and may suppress it. Likewise very slow consumption is also not advised as it doesn't achieve satiety and disturbs digestion. It is advised not to talk or laugh but to concentrate on food while eating. The diet consumed, considering the above facts get properly digested and maintains the health. Here are some simple rules, which are usually overlooked:

- The surroundings in which one eats should be pleasant and clean. The room should have adequate light and ventilation.
- The utensils used for cooking and eating should be clean.
- Personal hygiene should be maintained.
- Food should not be consumed in an angry, anxious or disturbed mood.
- The person who cooks the food should do so with love and affection in a pleasant state of mind.
- Eating should be a ritual and after eating one should show gratitude towards the person who has prepared the food.
- Food should not be taken atleast 3 hours before exercise and 1 hour after exercise.

Some seasonal changes should be made in the quantity and timings of food. e.g. the sun sets earlier in winter and also the appetite is stronger in winter. Hence the quantity of food should be increased according to the appetite and also the food timings should be earlier.

There are some definitions given in Ayurveda:

Adhyashana: Repeated eating or frequent eating of food i.e., to eat before the previous meal is digested is termed as adhyashana. The indications for digestion are a feeling of lightness of body, clear and odourless belch, excretion of stool and urine, etc.

Anashana: Consumption of food in a less quantity or not at all is termed as anashana. Anashana is recommended in various digestive disorders.

Contraindicated Food

The wrong combinations of food which vitiate doshas in such a manner that they act as toxins for the body are termed as Viruddha-aahar and are strongly contraindicated. These combinations are antagonistic to the properties of seven dhatus. The following factors are taken into account in context with 'viruddha-aahar'.

Desh viruddha: Desh can be taken as the land as well as the human body. e.g. dry, light and cold diet in jangal desh is antagonistic.

- Kaal viruddha: This is the diet antagonistic in context with time e.g., consumption of curds at night is prohibited.
- Agni viruddha: The food, which is ingested without understanding the capacity e.g., consumption of meat when digestive capacity is low.
- Matra viruddha: A mixture of foodstuffs mixed in a specific proportion may be toxic to the body e.g., consumption of ghee and honey in same proportion.
- Satmya viruddha: The food, which is not habitual, may cause harm e.g., intake of curds if not habitual may lead to disturbance of kapha dosha.
- Dosha viruddha: Intake of vata dominant food (dry, light, cold etc.) in an individual with vitiation of vata dosha may be harmful.
- Sanskar viruddha: Some foodstuffs if processed in a particular manner may turn toxic e.g., heating honey is contraindicated.
- Veerya viruddha: The mixture of two ingredients with opposite veerya (i.e., potency - hot & cold) is antagonist to the body e.g., combination of fish (hot) and milk (cold).
- Avastha viruddha: The diet consumed, which is, hot in accordance with the stage either of age or a disease is harmful e.g., in the severe stage of diarrhoea, ripen banana should be avoided.
- Kram viruddha: Ayurveda explains dietetic and behavioural regimen in sequence. Anything, which disturbs the sequence, is antagonistic. e.g. food taken without prior defaecation, micturition, feeling of hunger is harmful to the body.
- Parihar viruddha: Ayurveda recommends a specific dietary and behavioural regimen after any Panchakarma procedure or during treatment of any disease. The treatment is not fruitful if the regimen is not followed.
- Pak viruddha: Consuming properly cooked food is beneficial to the body. Improperly, partially cooked food is antagonistic e.g., improperly cooked rice can not be digested.
- Sanyoga viruddha: The food stuffs if taken separately do no harm but at the same time if mixed together act antagonistically e.g., any citrus fruit mixed with milk is contraindicated.
- Hrud viruddha: One should not take the food for which the person has apathy.

- Sampad viruddha: The food should be consumed in its original taste. The food with any change in its originality either because of fermentation or over ripening should not be consumed.

The diet consumed without considering the above principles may lead to disorders of skin, eyesight etc. We have listed some of the contraindicated food stuffs as follows:

1. Honey + Hot water
2. Honey + Ghee in same proportion
3. Honey in the person with aggravated pitta dosha.
4. Sour fruits with milk.
5. Black gram. Horse gram, pomegranate, coconut, Indian gooseberry, jackfruit, lemon, jejuba etc. should not be consumed with milk.
6. Radish, green leafy vegetables and garlic should not be consumed with milk.
7. All kinds of fishes with milk.
8. Milk mixed with curds.
9. Curds should not be heated.
10. Leaves of sesame plant should not be eaten.
11. Cow's flesh is strictly prohibited.
12. Vasa (unctuousness of fat) of buffalo and aquatic animals.
13. Pippali (Piper longum), common salt, chitrak (Plumbago zeylanica), bhallatak (Semicarpus anacardium) and kshar are prohibited in regular excess amount.
14. Salts with milk are to be avoided.

Thus these few examples will guide you towards a healthy life by keeping bodily constituents in equilibrium.

Digestion Physiology

Digestion is a process in which agni converts complex ingested food into such a form that can be easily assimilated in the body. Digestion plays a very important role in maintaining the health, by juvenating the bodily constituents viz. dosha, dhatu and mala. The whole focus of this Ayurvedic nutrition is to enhance the digestion.

Aaharchatushtay (four forms of aahar):

1. Bhakshya (food in the chewable form)
2. Bhojya (food in the eatable form)
3. Lehya (food which is licked)
4. Peya (food which is to be drunk)

The food is taken in the above four forms.

Now we will discuss the actual process of digestion, which takes place in two stages:

I. Sthoola Pachan
II. Sookshma Pachan

I. Sthoola Pachan (Gross digestion)

The food ingested gets churned by the teeth. Tongue along with bodhak kapha gives a bolus form to the food. Bodhak kapha is mainly responsible for understanding the taste. This bolus then reaches Aamashay with the help of Pranvayu, a type of vata dosha. (According to Sushrut Samhita).

Main role in further digestive process is carried out by Saman vayu. Kledak kapha - a subtype of kapha dosha lies in the upper portion of aamashay. The food in the bolus form now mixes with the kledak kapha and loses its solid state. Kledak kapha is sweet in taste, cool and semi-liquid in nature. Hence this 1st stage of digestion is termed as 'Madhur avasthapak'.

Pachak pitta - a subtype of pitta dosha lies in the lower portion of aamashay. After the first stage the food reaches the lower portion of aamashay where pachak pitta acts on it. The sweet taste of partly digested food from the first stage is converted to sour taste. And, this stage is termed as 'Amla avasthapak'. This partly digested food reaches pachak pitta in grahani. The sour taste of partly digested food from the second stage is converted to pungent taste by agni (jatharagni), the digestive capacity of pachak pitta. This is the third stage termed as 'Katu avasthapak'.

After these three stages, the digested material is divided by saman vayu into:

1. Saar - essence which is necessary for the replenishing and juvenation of bodily constituents.
2. Kitta - waste products

Taking the above description into consideration there are two school of thoughts. One of which gives importance to the site while the other emphasises on the action of agni.

1. Those who have given emphasis on the action of agni have given an illustration- while cooking rice in a pan, rice grains along with water get heated and eventually the mixture turns foamy - first stage. In the second stage, rice grains start becoming tender. And in the third stage the rice gets properly cooked to attain '*paripinditatwa*' (solid enough to be shaped into balls).
2. The other school of thought which emphasises on the site states that physiologically madhur rasa (sweet) lies above the level of aamashay and hence giving importance to the site the madhur - avasthapak.

Amla rasa (sour) is predominant in the region between aamashay and umbilicus, hence amla avasthapak.

Similarly katu rasa (pungent) is predominant below the level of umbilicus and so due to influence of this site, the third stage of digestion is of katu avasthapak. Though there are two different school of thoughts, digestion is a combination of both.

II. **Sookshma Pachan** (Minute Digestion)

Charak Samhita states: After the digestion by agni the aahar rasa (saar) formed is taken to the heart from where it is circulated throughout the body by vyan vayu (a subtype of vata dosha). This aahar rasa generates and replenishes the dhatus (bodily constituents) while circulation. Each dhatu has its own digestive capacity like jatharagni described in the digestion physiology, which is called dhatvagni. All these dhatvagr the derivatives of jatharagni.

The generation of dhatus takes place in an ideal sequence described below:

Rasa -> Rakta -> Mansa -> Meda -> Asthi -> Majja -> Shukra.

To explain this sequence there are three laws called as Nyay.

1. Kshirdadhi Nyay: Milk completely changes its form to curds when a little quantity of curd is added to milk. In the same manner rasa dhatu traverses to the site of rakta

dhatu and it completely changes itself to rakta dhatu. Similarly raktadhatu traverses to the site of mansa dhatu and gets converted to mansa dhatu; and so on.

2. Kedarkulya nyay: This law states that a small part of rasa dhatu nourishes the next dhatu rakta. A small part of rakta nourishes mansa and so on. This is well explained by giving an illustration of channelised watering in the agricultural farms.
3. Khale kapot Nyay: Khale kapot nyay is an analogy for a situation we see in the macrocosm. Birds from different places come to the site of food grains and after collecting the grains fly off to their respective places.

Among these three laws 'Kedarkulya nyay' is most commonly accepted.

Digestive Organs

The digestion takes place in the entire alimentary canal. Ayurveda sees the anatomy from different angle. It emphasises on physiology of digestion more than anatomy of digestive organs. They are:

1. Aamashay: This is the organ where food stays for a certain period of time in the partly digested stage. This can be taken as stomach and a part of duodenum.
2. Grahani: This is the part of small intestine which commences just after the aamashay and ends in pakvashay (large intestine). This can be taken as small intestine from the last part of duodenum to the ileocecal joint.
3. Pakvashay: This is that part of intestine where digested food stays for certain period of time. This can be taken as large intestine.

RECIPES

Sweet Dishes

Basundi

Ingredients:

Milk	4 lit.
Sugar	1 ¼ kg
Saffron	3 tablespoons
Cardamom powder	2 tablespoons
Nutmeg powder	2 tablespoons
Pistachio pieces	125 gms.

Benefits:

It increases kapha and is useful for vata and pitta dosha.

Caution:

Stir the milk properly while boiling.

Method of preparation:

1. Boil the milk in pan on low flame for about 1 hour and 50 minutes i.e., till the milk becomes thick.
2. Stir the milk while boiling.
3. Then add sugar, cut pieces of pistachio pieces in it.
4. Make the saffron slightly hot on flame & then crush it and mix it with little amount of milk and then add it to the basundi. Boil it for further 10 minutes.
5. Turn off the gas.
6. Serve cold or warm.

Note for better taste:

You can eat it with chapati or puri. While serving add cardamom & nutmeg powder to it.

Caramel Custard

Ingredients:

Milk	2 cups
Sugar	3 tablespoons
Water	1/2 cup
Eggs	3
Vanilla essence	1/2 teaspoon

Benefits:

This delicious dish nourishes the mind and body due to its soothing nature.

Caution:

Should not be consumed in diabetic and obese patients.

Method of preparation:

1. Heat a small saucepan on low flame.
2. Add sugar and water to it.
3. Bring to boil until the sugar dissolves in the water on a high flame.
4. Pour the caramel in a mould of one litre and keep aside.
5. Boil milk in a pan and let it become lukewarm.
6. Beat the eggs with the milk. Add the vanilla essence and sugar and milk. Stir well till the sugar dissolves completely.
7. Now pour this mixture in the earlier moulded mixture. Cover the mould properly with an aluminium foil.
8. Add the remaining water to a pressure pan. Place a steel net at the bottom of the pan. Keep the mould on the steel net.
9. Cover the pan with a lid and pressurise on a high flame. Lower the flame and cook for 10 minutes.
10. Then let the pan cool down. Remove the mould from the pressure pan and refrigerate for some time.
11. The custard is ready to serve for 6 persons.

Note for better taste:

Other essence can be added to get the flavour of your choice.
Serve chilled.

Garden Cress Seed Ladu (haliv seed)

Ingredients:

Seeds of garden cress	500 gms
Grated coconut	600 gms
Crushed jaggery	500 gms
Cardamom & nutmeg powder	2 teaspoons each
Coconut water	50 ml
Eatable gum resin	50 gms

Benefit:

Increases kapha and pitta. Reduces vata. Good for increasing breast milk. These seeds are high in proteins. Coconut reduces fatigue.

Method of preparation:

1. Soak garden cress seeds in coconut water for 30 minutes.
2. Mix all ingredients thoroughly except cardamom and nutmeg powder.
3. Keep mixture as it is for one hour.
4. Heat the mixture on low fire in a non-stick fry pan for 15-20 minutes. Stir well.
5. Remove from the flame and add cardamom and nutmeg powder.
6. Make lemon size balls.

Note for better taste:

Serve with hot milk.

Gulabjam

Ingredients:

Khoya	250 gm
Sugar	500 gm
Water	500 ml
Oil	200 ml

Benefit:

This sweat dish is very palatable and helps to achieve satiety.

Caution:
Individuals suffering from Grahani or Prameha should not consume it.

Method of preparation:

1. Intitially sugar syrup is prepared by keeping mixture of sugar and water on low flame. The mixture should be stirred constantly.
2. Sugar syrup becomes ready when the whole amount of sugar gets dissolved.
3. Khoya is made into small lemon sized balls. If required small amount of water or milk is added to it.
4. Frying pan with oil is kept on low flame.
5. These balls of khoya are deep-fried in the oil till they turn brown.
6. Fried balls are then allowed to cool and then kept in sugar syrup for about an hour.
7. And the sweet Gulab jams are ready to serve.

Note for better taste:

Cardamom powder and raisins can be mixed to khoya for better taste.

Moong Dal Flour Ladu (green gram flour sweet balls)

Ingredients:

Moong flour (green gram flour)	600 gms
Grind sugar	500 gms
Ghee	400 gms
Yellow raisins	100 gms
Cardamom powder	2 teaspoons

Benefit:

Good for vata and pitta. Increases kapha. Aged persons can also eat as they are easy to digest and very nutritious.

Caution:

Keep these ladus (sweet balls) in an airtight container. They remain delicious for one month.

Method of preparation:

1. Heat the ghee on low flame.
2. Add green gram flour to it.
3. Fry it for 20 minutes till it becomes golden yellow and gives aroma. Then turn off the gas.
4. Add sugar, yellow resins and cardamom powder.
5. Mix well and make the big lemon size balls.
6. Requires 30 minutes and nearly 25-30 balls can be prepared.
7. Same method can be used for preparing *besan* (chick peas flour) ladu, which are good for vata and increase kapha and pitta.

Rasala

Ingredients:

Curds from buffalo's milk drained of water content	1.25 Kg.
Sugar candy	1/2 Kg.
Powders of clove, cardamom, camphor and black pepper	1/2 teaspoon
Milk	2.5 lit.

Benefits:

It alleviates vata and pitta dosha. This is the best appetiser and an aphrodisiac beverage. It gives strength; relieves thirst, burning sensation and common cold. Especially recommended in Greeshma (summer) and Sharad (autumn).

Method of preparation:

1. Curds of buffalo's milk are taken.
2. It is kept in a bag of cotton cloth in such a way that the whole water content is drained out.
3. This curds without water is taken in the prescribed quantity.
4. Sugar candy in powdered form is added to the above curds.
5. The mixture is mashed in a way to make it homogeneous.
6. The milk is then added to this mixture and stirred well.
7. Cardamom, clove, camphor, black pepper in powdered form are added to the mixture.
8. And the Rasala is ready to serve.

Caution:

Rasala is not recommended in Vasant (spring) as it may increase kapha dosha.

Note for better taste:

Tastes better when served cold.

Shatavari Kalpa

Ingredients:

Sugar	1 kg
Shatavari roots	100 gm
Water (2 glasses)	400 ml
Sugar	400 gm
Cardamom (Velchi)	10 gm

Method of preparation:

1. Wash the roots thoroughly. Soak them overnight in the water. In the morning when the roots get swollen remove the skin and the central thread like portion.
2. Add about 1.25 litres of water to the middle fleshy portion. Boil it till we get a glassful 200 ml. of decoction. Filter it.
3. Add sugar and stir to form thick soup. Switch off the flame.
4. Add cardamom powder. Stir vigorously to form the granules.

Dose: 2-3 tablespoons preferably with milk.

Benefits:

This is a general tonic for all ages and good for the growth of the muscles. Useful for under nourished, retarded children. Promotes sleep by relieving from fatigue. Useful in psychosomatic disorders, epilepsy, and hysterics. Good for eyes, useful for computer operators, field workers, truck drivers, lab-technicians dealing with microscopes workers exposed to fumes, smoke, dust, direct heat, bright light, fire, etc. Good for the growth of the foetus as well for the pregnant women, used widely as galactogogue i.e. for promoting lactation. Summer tonic, cool in nature hence is more useful during summer. A tonic for the reproductive system of either sex found useful in menorrhagia. Useful in burning micturition, haematuria etc. found useful in-patients having urinary calculi. Useful in bleeding and non-bleeding piles, chronic constipation, blood stained stools, peptic and duedenal ulcers, hyperacidity, excessive perspiration, colitis, and long-standing mild fever.

Caution:

Sugar should be added in the appropriate proportion to avoid the loss of essential nutritives.

Note for better taste:
It is advised to consume with milk as a health drink.

Sheera (sweet cooked cream of wheat)

Ingredients:

Cream of wheat/ rava/ soji	250 gm
Water	400 ml
Milk	100 ml
Ghee	4 tablespoons
Bananas (chopped)	4
Sugar	200 gms
Saffron	1/4 teaspoon
Cardamom powder	1 teaspoon
Almonds (chopped)	10
Yellow raisins	20 pieces

Benefit:

Good for vata and pitta. Increases kapha. Dry fruits added to the dish gives taste and nutrition. Cardamom powder adds aroma to the dish.

Caution:

One should not use kapha increasing snacks containing excessive sweets. It is advisable to use warm drinks and spicy snacks in the morning.

Method of preparation:

1. Roast the cream of wheat in a non-stick pan for 5-10 minutes by adding ghee.
2. Add boiled water.
3. Cook for 10 minutes.
4. While cooking stir well.
5. Add boiled milk.
6. Cook for 5 minutes, stir well.
7. Add sugar and all other ingredients except cardamom powder. Keep the heavy lid on vessels and cook for 10 minutes.
8. Add cardamom powder while serving the dish.

Wholemeal Halwa

Ingredients:

Whole meal flour	250 gms
Sugar	200 gms
Ghee	25 gms
Ground cardamom	5 gms
Chopped pistachio nuts	1 tablespoon
Water	500 ml.

Benefits:

Balances tridoshas; gives strength.

Method of preparation:

1. Place sugar and water in a large pan.
2. Boil the mixture over a medium heat.
3. Then reduce heat and simmer for 5 minutes.
4. Melt ghee in a heavy based saucepan.
5. Add flour, sugar, water and cook.
6. Stir constantly until water evaporates and flour becomes soft.

Caution:

Diabetic patients should not take this recipe.

Milk Shakes/ Lassi/ Squash

Butter Milk

Ingredients:

Curds	250 gms
Water	1 litre

Benefit:

Appetiser, gives strength to intestine, and thus helps in irritable bowel syndrome.

Caution:

Don't add too much water or too less water to the curds.

Method of Preparation:

1. Take curds in an earthen pot. Add water to the curds.
2. Mix it thoroughly with a blender till it becomes homogeneous.
3. Buttermilk is ready to serve.

Note for Better Taste:

Asafoetida and salt can be added as per the taste.
Garnishing can be done with chopped coriander leaves.

Dhanyakpanak

Ingredients:

Coriander seeds	10 gms
Water	250 ml
Sugar	1 teaspoon
Camphor powder	1/4 teaspoon

Benefit:

Alleviates pitta dosha, relieves burning sensation, relieves burning micturation.

Caution:

Keep the preparation in an earthen pot.

Method of preparation:

1. Grind coriander seeds to the powder form.
2. Add sugar and camphor powder to the water. Stir well.
3. Add this water to the powdered coriander.
4. Strain the mixture to get a clear dhanyakpanak.

Note for better taste:

Rock salt can be added for taste.

Grape Wine

Ingredients:

Grape juice	1 litre
Flowers of Madhuca indica	5

Method of preparation:

1. Grape juice is kept in an earthen pot.
2. Flowers of Madhuca indica are added to the juice.
3. The pot is tightly closed at the brim with a piece of cloth.
4. The pot is kept in a dry and cool place for 21 days.
5. After 15 days the gas liberated is allowed to escape.
6. After 21st day the wine prepared can be taken out and served.

Benefits:

It is a good appetiser and digestive, releives thirst; beneficial in constipation. Acts as an aphrodisiac.

Caution:

Should be consumed with healthy and nutritious diet otherwise may vitiate doshas.

Note for better taste:

Barley with water or wheat with water can be kept with the flowers of Madhuca indica to prepare the wines of respective grains.

Gruel

Ingredients:

Rice grain	50 gm
Water	300 ml.

Method of preparation:

1. Wash and drain the rice properly.
2. Add water to the rice and keep it on a low flame.
3. Allow it to cook till the rice grains become tender (approximately 15 minutes).
4. After the rice is cooked more portion of liquid alongwith a very small portion of cooked is used for dietary purposes.

Benefits:

This helps to alleviate vata dosha. It also improves appetite hence can be given during and after any ailment. Gruels are also recommended in dietary regimen after panchakarma procedures.

Caution:

Care should be taken that water does not evaporate completely.

Note for better taste:

A pinch of pepper powder and rock salt can be added.

When the quantity of water is increased to 14 times, it is termed as 'mand'. Similarly if the quantity of water is reduced to 4 times, it is termed as 'vilepi'. Vilepi is comparatively thicker and heavier to digest.

Lemonade

Ingredients:

Freshly prepared lemon juice	50 ml.
Sugar water	300 ml.
Clove powder	1/4 teaspoon

Benefits:

This tasty juice is a good appetiser and digestive. It alleviates vata and pitta doshas.

Caution:

Use freshly prepared juice otherwise it vitiates pitta dosha.

Method of preparation:

All the ingredients in above proportion are mixed thoroughly.

Note for better taste:

Rock salt can be added to it.

Masala Milk

Ingredients:

Milk	250 ml.
A mixture of cardamom powder, nutmeg powder, dry ginger powder, in equal proportions	1/4 teaspoon
Saffron to garnish	1 pinch
Sugar	1 teaspoon

Benefits:

It alleviates vata and pitta doshas and increases kapha. It is a good aphrodisiac.

Caution:

Should not be consumed when digestive capacity is low.

Method of preparation:

Preheated cold milk is taken in a glass. The powders are added. Stir well. Then sugar is added as per the taste and saffron is sprinkled to garnish.

Note for better taste:

Honey can be added instead of sugar. Pieces of pistachio, cashew and almond can be added. If honey is added; the milk should be cold. If honey is heated; it becomes poison and desturbes the body.

Poppy Milk Shake

Ingredients:

Poppy seeds	1 teaspoon
Buffalo's milk	250 ml.
Cardamom	1/8 teaspoon
Nutmeg	1/8 teaspoon
Sugar	1 teaspoon

Benefits:

Alleviates vata dosha, increases kapha dosha, releives insomnia (recommended before going to bed).

Method of preparation:

1. Poppy seeds are soaked in buffalo's milk for four hours.
2. Cardamom and nutmeg powders are added and it is mixed well.
3. Sugar is added as per the taste.
4. The milk is allowed to cool and is then served with garnishing by pistachionuts.

Note for better taste:

The mixture can be heated and the milk is reduced and can be served hot.

Caution:

Individuals with low digestive capacity should consume it with dry ginger powder.

Raw Mango Crush

Ingredients:

Unripe mangoes	2
Mustard seeds	1/2 teaspoon
Asafoetida powder	1/4 teaspoon
Cow's ghee	1/2 teaspoon
Water	1 litre
Rock salt to taste	

Benefits:

Alleviates vata, alleviates doshas in the throat, reduces stammering; acts as a good appetiser, palatable.

Caution:

Intake of this crush in excess may vitiate pitta dosha.

Method of preparation:

1. Fry asafoetida powder in cow's ghee for two minutes.
2. Crush and make pulp of unripe mangoes.
3. Mix rock salt, mustard seeds, fried asafoetida powder with the pulp.
4. Add water to the mixture and blend it gently and the crush is ready to serve.

Note for better taste:

Pulp can be prepared by steaming the mangoes. Sugar can also be added for better taste.

Sharkarodak

Ingredients:

Sugar	2 tablespoons
Cardamom powder	1/4 teaspoon
Clove powder	1/4 teaspoon
Camphor powder	1/4 teaspoon
Black pepper	1/6 teaspoon
Water	500 ml.

Benefits:

Alleviates vata and pitta doshas. It is tasty, light and soothing in nature. It relieves fatigue, giddiness, and burning sensation.

Caution:

Black pepper should be added with caution so that the taste is not disturbed.

Method of preparation:

Mix all the ingredients thoroughly. And sweet sharkarodak is ready to drink.

Note for better taste:

Rock salt can be added. It can be added as a base syrup for various juices like lemon squash, mango-steen squash etc.

Tamarind Squash

Ingredients:

Tamarind	100 gm
Water	500 ml
Sugar	100 gm
Black pepper	1/4 teaspoon
Clove powder	1/8 teaspoon
Camphor powder	1/8 teaspoon

Benefits:

It alleviates vata dosha. It may increase pitta and kapha dosha. This is a good appetiser.

Method of preparation:

1. Ripen tamarind is soaked in water for about two hours.
2. The tamarind is mashed to make a pulp from it.
3. Sugar, pepper powder, clove, camphor are added to the mixture.
4. The mixture is then drained to get sweet and sour 'Tamarind squash'.

Caution:

This squash is not recommended in Sharad (Autumn) and Vasant (spring) seasons as it may increase pitta and kapha.

Note for better taste:

Rock salt can be added. Jaggery can be used instead of sugar.

Miscellaneous

Paan

Ingredients:

Betel leaves	2
Betel nut (circular pieces)	3
Saturated solution of limestone with water	1/12 teaspoon
Saturated solution of Acacia catechu powder with water	1/8 teaspoon
Ginger paste	1/8 teaspoon
Musk, Camphor, Saffron & Grated dried coconut	125 mg each
Mace & Nutmeg powder	60 mg each
Sweet root, Cinnamon, & Fennel seeds	125 mg each
Almond pieces	1/2
Clove & Cardamom	1 each
Dry ginger powder, Tailed pepper & Helix aspera	125 mg each

Benefits:
Offering paan is friendly gesture and custom in India. Paan has pungent, bitter, sweet taste and is hotting potent. It alleviates vata and kapha. It is a wonderful mouth freshener and removes bad odour of mouth. It also acts as a wormicidal and an aphrodisiac preparation. It is beneficial in diabetes and urinary disorders.

Method of preparation:
1. Saturated solutions of limestone and Acacia catechu are prepared in water. Both the solutions are kept aside.
2. Two betel leaves are taken. The point of the apex and base are cut.
3. Saturated solution of limestone is applied to one of the leaves with the thumb.
4. Then catechu solution is applied.
5. Both the solutions are mixed homogeneously on the leaf.
6. Rests of the ingredients are added one by one.
7. The other leaf is kept below the first one and both the leaves are folded in such a fashion that all the ingredients get covered properly.
8. Silver foil is then applied over the 'paan' and is then offered with affection.

Note for better taste:
Gulkand (jelly made from rose petals), cherry, etc. can be added to the ingredients.

Caution:
Paan with, catechu in excess is anaphrodisiac.
Paan should never be consumed just after intake of milk.
It is advised to spit out first salivary secretions as they may vitiate the doshas.

Spicy Tea

Ingredients:

Milk	250 ml.
Water	250 ml.
Teabags	2
Ginger	5 gm
Green cardamoms	2-3
Saffron	2 sticks
Sugar to taste.	

Benefits:

Relieves fatigue, appetiser, balances tridoshas.

Caution:

Ginger should not be added to this tea in greeshma (summer) rutu.

Method of preparation:

1. Put water and milk together in a saucepan.
2. Boil the mixture. Add the teabags, cardamoms, ginger (crushed), saffron and sugar to it.
3. Lower the heat.
4. Bring slowly back to the boil and boil for 3-5 minutes.
5. Strain into a teapot and discard the spices. The tea is ready to serve.

Note for better taste:

Can be served with or without sugar. This beverage can be served after a meal.

Tea

Ingredients:

Lemongrass leaves	30 gm
Basil leaves	30 gm
Dry ginger piece	10 gm
Cinnamon sticks	2
Sugar	2 teaspoon
Water	700 ml.

Benefits:

Alleviates kapha and vata; beneficial in fever, fatigue, body ache, chills etc.

Caution:

In summer (greeshma), it is not recommended.

Method of preparation:

1. Basil leaves and lemongrass leaves are cut into small pieces.
2. All the ingredients are mixed and kept on low flame.
3. The water is reduced to half.
4. The decoction prepared is served hot.

Note for better taste:

In winter dry ginger can be increased as per the taste.
Mint leaves can also be added to the mixture.

Sauce

Peanuts Sauce

Ingredients:

Peanuts	100 gms
Spring onions	3
Honey	2 teaspoons
Soya sauce	1 teaspoons
Water	1 cup
Garlic	4 cloves
Coconut cream	2 teaspoons
Red chilly powder	1 teaspoons
Salt to taste	

Benefits:

Increases pitta and kapha.
High in proteins.

Method of preparation:

1. Combine all ingredients except coconut cream in a blender.
2. Blend it till smooth.
3. Keep a pan on low flame.
4. Add the blended mixture to the pan and cook over for 5 minutes till the sauce thickens.
5. Cool it, and then add the coconut cream.

Note for better taste:

This dish can be served with plain rice.

Toast/ Roast/ Sandwich

Bread Sandwich

Ingredients:

Slices of bread	4
Butter (salted will do)	6 teaspoons
Green coconut chutney	6 teaspoons
Sliced cucumber	1
Sliced tomato	1
Cumin seed powder	2 teaspoons
Salt as per taste	

Benefit:

Easy to prepare and easy to digest.

Caution:

Do not add too much of salt.

Method of Preparation:

1. Apply butter to all the slices of bread.
2. Next apply the chutney above the layer of butter to all the slices.
3. Lay one-two slices of cucumber and tomato each on 2 slices of bread.
4. Sprinkle salt and cumin seed powder over it.
5. Cover these 2 slices by the remaining 2 slices of bread and the sandwiches are ready to serve.

Note for Better Taste:

Many other vegetables can be added to the sandwich.
These sandwiches can be roasted in a toaster for good taste.
They can be served with different types of sauces.

Pakoras (Speciality of Indian food, can be prepared from any vegetables)

Onion Pakora

Ingredients:

Chick flour	250 gms
Onion	1
Chilli powder	2 teaspoons
Sesame oil	250 ml
Turmeric powder	1 teaspoon
Salt to taste	
Water to make paste	

Benefit:

Reduces vata. Increases kapha and pitta.

Caution:

Don't add baking powder to make it crispy by which it is heavy to digest.

Method of preparation:

1. Chop the onions in vertical plane.
2. Mix the chick flour, turmeric powder and salt in a bowl.
3. Stir gradually by adding sufficient (less) water so as to prepare thick batter consistency.
4. Heat the oil in a frying pan.
5. Take onion pieces and dip them in the paste and put these pieces one by one in the hot oil.
6. Deep-fry this mixture till it changes its colour to golden brown.
7. Drain on an absorbent paper.

Note for better taste:

Serves for 4-5 persons. Served with sauce or chutney (paste of coriander, grated coconut, green chillies, ginger and salt to taste).

In the same way onion can be replaced by potatoes, brinjals, spinach, cauliflower, capsicum etc. to make respective pakoras.

Vermicelli Porridge

Ingredients:

Vermicelli	100 gms
Milk	1 lit.
Ghee	2 teaspoons
Sugar	12-13 teaspoons
Chopped and Cashew nuts	2 teaspoons each
Almonds	2 teaspoons
Yellow raisin	2 teaspoons
Saffron	½ teaspoons
Cardamom powder	2 teaspoons
Hot water	1 cup

Benefits:

It increases kapha dosha and it is good for vata & pitta dosha.

Caution:

Roast the vermicelli carefully in ghee on low flame. Roast it till it turns slight brown.

Method of preparation:

1. Crush the vermicelli.
2. Roast it in ghee on low flame till they turn slight brown.
3. Add hot water in it and boil it in water till it gets tender.
4. Remove the excess water.
5. Then add milk into vermicelli and again boil it in milk.
6. Take the saffron in a bowl and make it slightly hot on low flame and then crush it and add a teaspoon of milk in it and mix it thoroughly.
7. Remove the porridge from the burner and then add sugar, cashew nut, almonds, raisins and saffron to it and stir it well. Add cardamom powder to it.

Note for better taste:

You can eat this with chapati or puri. You can make wheat porridge, rice porridge, carrot porridge, and sago porridge with the same recipes.

Chutney/ Raita

Brinjal Raita

Ingredients:

Large flowered byronica (Coccinia indica)	100 gm
Brinjal (approx.)	250 gm (approximately)
Ginger paste	1/2 teaspoon
Garlic paste	1/2 teaspoon
Black pepper powder	1/4 teaspoon
Asafoetida	1/4 teaspoon
Cumin seeds powder	1/2 teaspoon
Buttermilk	100 ml.
Rock salt to taste	

Benefits:

Alleviates kapha dosha, beneficial in obesity, diabetes etc.

Caution:

Not recommended in hyperacidity.

Method of preparation:

1. Brinjal is first roasted until it turns black.
2. The outer skin of brinjal is removed to get the pulp of brinjal.
3. Byronica is cut into small pieces.
4. Pulps of brinjal, pieces of byronica garlic paste, ginger paste are mixed together.
5. Buttermilk is added to the mixture.
6. Spices are then mixed and raita is ready to serve.

Note for better taste:

Honey and mint leaves can be used to garnish the dish.

Curry Leaves Chutney (paste/ powder)

Ingredients:

Fresh curry leaves	100 gms
Grated dry coconut	100 gms
Sesame seeds	100 gms
Red chilli powder	3 teaspoons
Sugar powder	1 teaspoon
Oil	2 tablespoons
Salt to taste	

Benefit:

It increases pitta and reduces vata and kapha doshas.

Method of preparation:

1. Fry the curry leaves on hot oil for 5-10 minutes.
2. Roast the sesame seeds and dry coconut separately for 10 minutes each on a low flame.
3. Then put all the ingredients in a mixer and mix well.

Note for better taste:

It lasts for 10-20 days. You can mix curd to it. It enhances the taste. With the same recipe one can make chutney of sesame seeds and roasted groundnut.

Dates with Tamarind

Ingredients:

Dates (seedless)	200 gms.
Tamarind paste	100 gms.
Jaggery	100 gms.
Ground ginger	1 teaspoon
Ground coriander	1 teaspoon
Salt (rock salt)	1 teaspoon
Water	200 ml.

Benefits:

Balances tridoshas, gives strength, appetiser, relieves constipation, tastelessness ètc.

Caution:

Don't heat the ingredients as heating reduces the nutritive value.

Method of preparation:

1. Make a fine paste of all the above ingredients.
2. Transfer to a clean dry jar and cover it.

Note for better taste:

Sugar can be added instead of jaggery.

Fresh Mixed Herb Raitha

Ingredients:

Fresh mint leaves	50 gm
Fresh basil leaves	50 gm
Fresh dill leaves	50 gm
Fresh coriander leaves	50 gm
Natural yoghurt	150 gm
Water	50 ml.
Salt and sugar to taste	

Benefits:

Balances tridoshas.

Caution:

All the herbs should be taken fresh and the chopping should not be too fine.

Method of preparation:

1. Coarsely chop the herbs.
2. Place yoghurt and water in a bowl.
3. Whip until smooth.
4. Add all the herbs, sugar and salt to taste. Mix well and serve.

Note for better taste:

This dish can be served with roti, paratha or bread.

Grated Coconut Chutney

Ingredients:

Grated coconut	100 gms
Chopped coriander	50 gms
Cloves of garlic	10
Green chillies (cut into pieces)	4
Ginger	4 inch piece

Salt and sugar to taste.

Benefits:

It is good for vata and kapha dosha but it aggravates pitta dosha.

Method of preparation:

Take all the ingredients in mixer and blend them well. Chutney is ready.

Note for better taste:

You can eat this in your meal or you can apply it on bread and can make sandwiches. With the same recipe you can make chutney of garlic and coriander.

Green Chutney

Ingredients:

1. Mint leaves	50 gm
2. Garlic	05 gm
3. Dry ginger powder	1/4 teaspoon
4. Asafoetida	1/4 teaspoon
5. Pepper powder	1/4 teaspoon
6. Coriander leaves	50 gm
7. Lemon juice	10 ml.

Benefits:

This chutney is a very good appetiser and digestive preparation. Can be safely administered in irritable bowel syndrome, diarrhoea, and indigestion, giving strength to the intestine.

Method of preparation:

1. Mint leaves, coriander leaves, garlic are crushed to make a pulp form.
2. Powder of dry ginger, asafoetida, black pepper are added to the pulp and mixed well.
3. Lemon juice is then added to this preparation.

Note for better taste:

Buttermilk can be added instead of lemon juice to get liquid form to the chutney. Wood apple pulp can also be added to the chutney.

SOUPS

Soups are used as starters as they are light and healthy appetisers. A tremendous range of colours & textures can be used while preparing soups. Spices, herbs and garnishes add the final touch.

Carrot, Tomato & Cardomom Soup

Ingredients:

Cardamom pods	9
Fresh tomatoes	275 gms
Carrots	275 gms
Sesame oil	1 ½ teaspoons
Onion	1
Vegetable stock	975 ml

Salt & freshly ground pepper to taste
Fresh coriander or parsley for garnish

Benefits:

High in fibre from vegetables. Cardamom is a rich, aromatic spice that belongs to the ginger spice. Balances tridoshas. It is low in calories.

Caution:

Choose fresh green or white pods for this soup, as the small, dark seeds retain essential oils that are missing in ready – ground supplies.

Method of preparation: (Requires ½ hour)

1. Roughly crush the cardamom pods using a pestle & mortar.
2. Place all the pods & seeds in a piece of muslin & tie securely with a string.
3. Skin the tomatoes by plunging them into a bowl of hot water for 30 seconds. Cold for 1 minute, until the skins can be easily removed using ones fingers. Dressed the tomatoes, trim the carrots & roughly chop them both.
4. Heat the oil in a large saucepan and cook the chopped onion over a medium heat.
5. Add the carrots & tomatoes and cook for atleast 2-3 minutes.
6. Add the stock & wrapped cardamom pods, and bring to boil.
7. Reduce the heat & simmer for about 30 minutes until the carrots are tender.
8. Remove the cardamom from the pan & leave to cool; then squeeze the muslin out over the pan, extracting all the juices.
9. Puree the vegetables & their liquid & reheat gently.

Note for better taste:

Serve hot. Garnish with sprinkling of chopped coriander or parsley. You may like to try serving this soup with Indian breads, such as nan & paratha. For non- vegetarians instead of vegetable stock chicken stock can be used.

Mixed Vegetable Soup

Ingredients:

Cauliflower	150 gms
Carrot	150 gms
French beans	150 gms
Green peas	100 gms
Water	300 ml
Corn flour	2 teaspoons
Ghee/ sesame oil	1 teaspoon
Salt to taste	

Benefit:

High fibre content. Balances tridoshas.

Caution:

Don't chop the vegetables to very small pieces otherwise all essential nutrients will be lost.

Method of preparation:

1. Requires half an hour including preparation time.
2. Steams cook all the vegetables on low heat.
3. Add ghee/ oil in heated pan.
4. Add corn flour to the pan and saute till it becomes golden yellow.
5. Add boiling water to the pan and stir well for 5-10 minutes.
6. Add steamed vegetables and salt and serve.

Note for better taste:

Serve hot with chilli, soya sauce and black pepper powder.

Moong Dal Soup

Ingredients:

Yellow moong dal	100 gms
Water	300 ml
Ghee	2 teaspoons
Cumin seeds & Turmeric powder (curcuma)	1 teaspoon each
Coriander leaves	25 gms
Salt to taste	

Benefits:
Easy to digest.
Increases agni. Balances Tridoshas.

Caution:
Too much of salt reduces the effectiveness of the soup.

Method of preparation:
1. Wash & drain moong dal properly.
2. Keep ready the chopped coriander leaves.
3. Boil water.
4. In the boiling water add drained dal & turmeric powder.
5. Cook on low flame.
6. Melt ghee in another pan.
7. Add cumin seeds to ghee after it gets hot.
8. Let the seeds pop up.
9. Now add the dal. Stir it well.
10. Make a homogenous mixture.
11. Add salt to it.
12. The thickness of soup depends on you.

Note for better taste:

This soup can be served with coriander leaves garnishing it. Pieces of bread, fried in oil can be added to the soup or small amount of pepper can be added for taste by which Kapha dosha is reduced.

Mushroom Soup

Ingredients:

Flat or field mushrooms	400 gms
Medium onion	1/2
Carrot	1
Garlic	1 clove
Medium potato	1
Virgin olive oil	2 tablespoons
Bay leaf	1
Nutmeg powder	2 pinches

Juice of 1/2 lemon
Salt and white pepper to taste.
Benefit: High in fibre from vegetables. Low in calories. Balances tridoshas.

Method of preparation:

1. Chop the onion, garlic, carrot and dice the potato.
2. Heat the oil in a large frying pan.
3. Keep aside a few small mushrooms for the garnish.
4. Take the stalks off.
5. Add caps and stalks to the pan with onion, potato, carrot, garlic and bay leaf.
6. Cook for 10 minutes stirring constantly.
7. Add one litre water.
8. Simmer for 30 minutes and add nutmeg powder and lemon juice.
9. Blend the vegetable broth and reheat gently and serve.

Note for better taste:

Add the mushroom slices and serve.

Potato, Cabbage and Chilli Soup

Ingredients:

Small cabbage	1/2
Potatoes	250 gms
Red chilli powder	1/4 teaspoon
Onion	1 large size
Garlic	2 clove
Olive oil	2 tablespoon
Vegetable/ Chicken stock	1 litre
Fresh red chilli	1
Salt to taste	

Benefit:

Reduces kapha dosha. High in fibre from onion and cabbage. Reduces the risk of getting certain cancers. Ease high blood pressure.

Method of preparation:

1. Peel and finely chop onion, garlic and chilli.
2. Heat the olive oil in a large pan.
3. Add onion, garlic, chilli or chilli powder.
4. Cook on a high heat for 5 minutes.
5. Stir occasionally.
6. Dice the potatoes and add with 500 ml of the stock to the pan.
7. Cover and simmer for five minutes.
8. Wash the cabbage and cut it into pieces of one inch.
9. Add it to the pan.
10. Cover and steam for 10 minutes.
11. Add rest of stock, bring to the boil and simmer for 30 minutes.
12. Use a wooden spoon pressed against the side of the pan to break down the potatoes.

Note for Better Taste:

Add salt and pepper to taste and serve.

Pumpkin and White Bean Soup

Ingredients:

Dried white beans	225 gms
Small pumpkin	1
Onion & Bay leaf	1 each
Garlic	2 cloves
Vegetable or Chicken stock	1.5 lit
Dried thyme	1 ½ teaspoon
Semi- skimmed milk	450 ml
Ground black pepper & Paprika	½ teaspoon each
Celery leaves	
Salt to taste	

Benefits:
Reduces Kapha dosha and vitiates Pitta.

Caution:
Heat on low flame so that essential minerals are not lost.

Method of preparation:
(Requires 2 hrs)

1. Soak the beans in cold water.
2. Drain them & place in a large saucepan
3. Roughly chop the onion & garlic, add them to the pan with 1 lit. of stock, I teaspoon of dried thyme & bay leaf.
4. Bring to boil & then reduce heat. Cover & simmer for about 1 hr until the beans are tender.
5. Peel the pumpkin and discard the seeds.
6. Finely dice the flesh and simmer in the reserved stock & thyme for 15 minutes until tender.
7. Allow to cool, then remove the bay leaf from the beans, add pumpkin squash, milk, stock mixture and puree until smooth.
8. Return to the pan & heat gently.

Note for better taste:

Sprinkle paprika in the centre of each serving & garnish with chopped celery leaves. In North America, farmers grow a great range of squashes, including the succulent butternut variety, which could be substituted to pumpkin in recipe.

Spinach Soup

Ingredients:

Chopped Spinach	300 gms
Medium size onions	1
Mashed ginger	1 teaspoon.
Cloves of garlic	4
Ghee/ sesame oil	2 teaspoons
Medium size tomatoes	2
Salt to taste.	

Benefit:

Good for Pitta and Vata doshas.
High in fibre from spinach.
Can be used in chronic constipated patients.

Caution:

Serve it hot or it will be a burden to the digestion process.

Method of Preparation:

1. Melt the ghee/ sesame oil in a heated pan.
2. Add chopped onion and garlic to the ghee.
3. Saute on low fire till it becomes golden yellow.
4. Add spinach, ginger & tomatoes.
5. Cook for 10 minutes on low fire.
6. Add salt & puree the mixture.
7. Reheat the mixture & serve.

Note for better taste:

Grated cheese can be added to it. But if Kapha dosha is vitiated don't add cheese to the soup.

Tomato Soup

Ingredients:

Tomatoes	4
Chopped Green Chillies	2-3
Ghee	1 tablespoon
Cumin seeds	½ teaspoon
Asafoetida	¼ teaspoon
Salt to taste.	

Benefit:

It is a good appetiser, and easy to digest.

Method of Preparation:

1. Tomatoes are kept for boiling.
2. The skin is peeled off after boiling.
3. Ghee is heated in a preheated pan on a low flame.
4. Add cumin seeds, chillies, and asafoetida to the ghee.
5. Add the tomatoes to the pan and mash them.
6. Mix thoroughly.
7. The tomato soup is ready to serve.

Caution:

Salt should be added in less quantity.

Note for Better Taste:

Fried breadcrumbs can be added. Sugar can also be added as per the taste.

Watercress Soup

Ingredients:

Onion (small)	One
Potatoes	450 gms
Vegetable stock	500 ml
Semi skimmed milk	250 ml
Ground nutmeg	1/4 teaspoon
Lemon Juice	1 tablespoon
Natural Yoghurt	1 tablespoon
Watercress	2-3 bunches
Ground black pepper	1/2 teaspoon
Salt to taste	

Benefit:

Low in calories, fat, cholesterol and sodium. Increases kapha and reduces vata dosha.

Caution:

As watercress is highly perishable, buy it no more than one day before you intend to use it.

Method of preparation:

1. Chop the onion and dice the potatoes, then place them in a large saucepan with the stock, milk, and nutmeg.
2. Bring to the boil and reduce the heat.
3. Cover and simmer for 15-20 minutes until the potatoes are tender.
4. Choose fresh, bright green watercress with crisp leaves.
5. Wash them reserving a few springs for garnish.
6. Add the cress and lemon juice to the saucepan.
7. Remove from the heat immediately and allow to cool for a while.
8. Puree the mixture until smooth.
9. Return to the pan.
10. Reheat gently and serve.

Note for better taste:

Garnish with watercress leaves. Serve with lightly buttered toast fingers on the side. The peppery flavour of watercress lends itself well to soups, and this dish can be served hot or cold as a refreshing summer soup.

Vegetables

Boiled Potato Vegetable

Ingredients:

Potato	1/2 kg
Onion	1
Turmeric powder	1/2 teaspoon
Green chillies	2-3
Mustard seeds	1 teaspoon
Grated coconut	2-3 teaspoons
Sesame oil	2 teaspoons

Benefits:

Increases vata dosha.

Caution:

Boil the potatoes in a pressure cooker and not in an open pan.

Method of preparation:

1. Boil the potatoes for 25 minutes.
2. Peal off after cooling.
3. Cut the potatoes into small pieces.
4. Heat the oil in a pan on a low flame and add mustard seeds.
5. Let the seeds pop up and then add turmeric powder and asafoetida powder in it.
6. Add chopped green chillies.
7. Then add chopped onion to the pan and saute it till golden brown.
8. Then add chopped potatoes and saute it properly.
9. Keep it on a low flame for 5 minutes. Stir well.
10. Add salt and stir.
11. Off the gas and allow it to cool slightly.
12. Garnish it with grated coconut and chopped coriander leaves.

Note for better taste:

Serve hot. This vegetable is served with rotis or parathas. This vegetable can be cooked without prior boiling of potatoes.

Butter Milk Curry (Kadhi/ Matha)

This is also called buttermilk soup.

Ingredients:

Water	400 ml
Curds	100 gms
Ground turmeric	½ teaspoon
Cumin seeds	½ teaspoon
Curry leaves	2-4 leaves
Green chilli	1
Ginger	½ inch
Chicken pea flour	1 teaspoon
Sugar and salt to taste	

Benefits:

Balances Tridoshas.

Caution:

Curds should be freshly prepared.

Method of preparation:

1. Blend curds by adding water to it. Keep ready paste of ginger & chilli.
2. Heat the pan.
3. Add ghee and heat it.
4. Add cumin seeds and let them pop up.
5. Add asafoetida powder & pinch of turmeric (curcuma) powder along with curry leaves.
6. Add paste of ginger & chilli to it.
7. Now add blended curd i.e. butter milk in the pan & boil for 5 minutes.

Note for better taste:

Garnish by coriander leaves (chopped). Serve hot with plain rice. Bengal gram dal flour (1 teaspoon) can be added so that the soup becomes slight thick.

Cabbage Vegetable

Ingredients:

Fresh cabbage	500 gms
Green peas	100 gms
Coconut (grated)	2-3 teaspoons
Coriander leaves (chopped)	2-3 teaspoons
Green chillies	2
Sesame oil	2 teaspoons
Turmeric powder	1 teaspoon
Asafoetida powder	1/4 teaspoon
Salt to taste.	

Benefits:

Good for kapha and pitta.

Caution:

Don't chop the cabbage into very small pieces, otherwise all essential nutrients will be lost.

Method of preparation:

1. Wash the cabbage.
2. Chop into small pieces.
3. Heat oil in a frying pan on a low flame.
4. Add mustard seeds to the pan.
5. Let the seeds pop up.
6. Add green chillies, asafoetida powder, turmeric powder to the pan.
7. Then add chopped cabbage and green peas to the pan.
8. Saute well for 2-3 minutes.
9. Keep a lid on the pan and put some water on the lid.
10. Saute well repeatedly.
11. When the vegetable in the pan becomes tender, add salt and cook for 5 minutes.
12. Add coconut and coriander for garnishing after cooling.

Note for better taste:

Avoid reheating. Serve hot. Chopped potatoes can be added to it. Avoid giving this vegetable to patients having calculus.

Dal-Fry

Ingredients:

Red gram	200 gm
Mustard	¼ tablespoon
Turmeric	¼ tablespoon
Chopped coriander leaves	1 tablespoon
Curry leaves	7 leaves
Chooped chillies	2
Oil	1 tablespoon
Water	650 ml
Asafoetida	1 pinch
Salt to taste	

Benefit:

This is digestive, nourishing dish usually taken with roti or rice.

Caution:

Individuals suffering from hyperacidity should consume this dish in very less quantity.

Method of preparation:

1. Red grams are washed, rinsed and cooked with 400 ml of water till they become tender.
2. These tender red grams are blended coarsly with a blender.
3. Frying pan is kept on medium flame and the oil is added to it.
4. Mustard seeds are added to the oil. When they start popping turmeric and asafoetida areadded to the oil.
5. Curry leaves and chillies are then taken to the pan.
6. Tender red gram is added to the pan gently.
7. Remaining water alongwith salt is added to the pan and mixed gently.
8. Few coriander leaves are mixed with dal during preparation and few are kept to garnish.
9. Dal is allowed to boil for 3-5 minutes and then taken in a serving bowl.

Note for better taste:

Small amount of sugar and chopped tomatoes can be added to the dal.

Green Peas Vegetable

Ingredients:

Green peas	500 gms
Medium size onions	1
Oil	1 tablespoons
Grated coconut	2 tablespoons
Chopped coriander leaves	50 gms
Mustard seeds	1 teaspoon
Turmeric powder	1 teaspoon
Asafoetida powder	¼ teaspoon
Red chilli powder	2 teaspoons
Jaggery to taste.	
Salt to taste	

Benefit:

Increases vata and pitta. Balances kapha.

Method of preparation:

1. Chop the onions into small pieces.
2. Heat oil in a pan on low flame.
3. Add mustard seeds & let them pop up.
4. Then add asafoetida, turmeric powder, and red chilli powder to the oil.
5. Add chopped onions & fry it till golden brown.
6. Now add green peas.
7. Stir intermittently.
8. Cook on steam and if required add water.
9. When peas are tender add salt and jaggery and cook for 10 minutes.
10. Turn off the flame.
11. Garnish with grated coconut and coriander leaves.

Note for better taste:

This dish can be served with chapattis. In this way all type of beans can be cooked.

Green Spicy Curry

Ingredients:

Fresh lime juice	1 teaspoon
Grated coconut	4 tablespoons
Chopped coriander leaves	2 tablespoons
Green chillies	3-4
Fennel seeds	2 teaspoon
Cinnamon	2 sticks
Cardamom	3
Onions (chopped)	1
Potatoes, Carrot, & Clove	2 each
Green peas	1/2 cup
French beans	50 gm
Cauliflower	250 gm
Water	3 cups
Oil	3 tablespoons
Salt to taste	

Benefits:
Reduces kapha dosha.
Gives nutrition to the body.

Caution:
Spices should be added in proportion.

Method of preparation:
1. Add some water to the grated coconut and blend the mixture to get milk of coconut.
2. Make a paste of chopped onion, fennel seeds, chillies and coriander leaves.
3. Roast the cloves, cardamom, cinnamon together and grind it.
4. Heat a pressure pan. Add oil to it. Add the above paste to it.
5. Stir well. Chop the potatoes, carrots, french beans, and cauliflower.
6. Add the chopped vegetables along with green peas to the pan.
7. Stir constantly for 2-3 minutes.
8. Now add the powder of spices and salt to the above mixture. Again stir well.
9. Add milk of coconut and limejuice after the vegetables become tender.
10. Stir well and the recipe is ready to serve.

Note for better Taste:
This recipe can be served with rotis or rice.

Spicy Mixed Lentils

Ingredients:

Small yellow lentils (Green gram dal)	50 gms
Yellow split peas (Bengal gram dal)	50 gms
Red gram dal	50 gms
Turmeric powder	1/4 teaspoon
Ginger paste	1/4 teaspoon
Coriander seeds	1/4 teaspoon
Black mustard seeds	1/2 teaspoon
Cumin seeds	1/2 teaspoon
Dried curry leaves	8 - 10
Asafoetida	1/4 teaspoon
Green chillies	2
Edible oil	1-2 tablespoon
Fenugreek seeds	1/2 teaspoon
Salt to taste	

Benefits:
Alleviates vata dosha, highly nutritious, increases digestion.

Caution:
Contraindicated in persons having hyperacidity.

Method of preparation:

1. Wash and drain the lentils properly.
2. Then soak the lentils in water for half an hour.
3. Again drain the lentils and place in a pan with 300 ml. water, salt, 1/2 tablespoon oil and turmeric powder over a medium heat.
4. Bring to boil and then simmer for 10-15 minutes until the lentils become tender.
5. Then blend the mixture until smooth.
6. Finely chop the chillies.
7. Heat another large pan and add the remaining oil to the pan.
8. Add all the spices one by one and cook. Stir constantly for 1 minute.
9. Then add the blended lentil mixture and cook for 2-5 minutes.
10. Again add water (400 ml.) to the pan and bring to the boil.
11. Cook for 5 minutes and then the recipe is ready to serve for 2 persons.

Note for better taste: Other types of lentils can be added. Coriander leaves and grated coconut can be used for garnishing.

Spicy Tomato

Ingredients:

Onion (large)	1
Tomatoes	3
Ginger chopped	1 teaspoon
Green chillies	2
Ground coriander leaves	1 bunch
Turmeric powder	1/4 tablespoon
Whole bread	4-5
Oil	1 tablespoon
Cumin seeds	1/2 teaspoon
Salt to taste.	

Benefits:

Alleviates kapha dosha.

Caution:

Spices should be added with caution so as to avoid aggravation of pitta dosha.

Method of preparation:

1. Chop the onions, tomatoes and green chillies.
2. Heat oil in a saucepan.
3. Add onions, cumin seeds, ginger, chillies.
4. Stir frequently and cook for 10 minutes until colour of onions change to light golden.
5. Stir in tomatoes, cook for 5 minutes.
6. Add ground coriander, turmeric powder and salt and cook for 2 minutes.
7. Serve with bread.

Note for better taste:

Garnishing can be done by cashew nuts, pistachio nuts etc. Sugar can be added for taste.

Stuffed Lady Finger

Ingredients:

Lady finger	250 gms
Grated Coconut	4 teaspoons
Coriander (leaves)	50 gms
Red chilly powder	1 teaspoon
Sesame oil	2 teaspoons
Mustard seeds	10gms
Asafoetida powder	1gm
Turmeric powder	½ teaspoon
Groundnut powder	25gms
Salt to taste	

Benefits:

Increases pitta dosha.

Caution:

Don't add too much of spicy masala.

Method of preparation:

1. Wash and drain ladyfingers.
2. Wipe them with a cotton cloth.
3. Cut each vertically (halfway)
4. For making the stuff mix groundnut powder, red chilli powder, grated coconut, salt together.
5. Stuff each ladies finger with this mixture.
6. Meanwhile heat a pan and add oil to it.
7. Add mustard seeds. Let them pop up. Then add turmeric & asafoetida powder.
8. Add the vegetable to it. Sauté it for 3 minutes. Keep lid on the pan.
9. When it gets properly cooked i.e. it becomes tender, off the gas.
10. Serve hot.

Note for better taste:
Garnish with coriander leaves. Before adding vegetable to the pan, chopped onion can also be added to increase the taste.
In this way any stuffed vegetable can be made such as capsicum, tomatoes, brinjals etc.

Stuffed Tomatoes

Ingredients·

Small size tomatoes	5
Big onion	1
Grated coconut	4-5 teaspoons
Cloves	2-3 pieces
Black pepper powder	1 teaspoon
Red chilli powder & Turmeric powder	1 teaspoon each
Mustard seeds, & Cumin seeds	1 teaspoon each
Crushed groundnut powder	5-6 teaspoons
Asafoetida powder	½ teaspoon
Sesame oil	2-3 teaspoon
Ginger piece (fresh)	½ inch
Garlic	3-4 cloves
Jaggery to taste	
Salt to taste	

Benefits:
Good for kapha. Increases pitta dosha.

Caution:
Don't add too much of spicy masala or it will affect the digestion process.

Method for Preparation:

I. Mixture for stuffing the tomatoes
1. Make paste of ginger & garlic with grated coconut.
2. Chop onion into pieces. Roast the pieces on low flame till golden brown.
3. Make paste of onion with earlier paste.

II. Put the pan on low flame and heat the oil.
1. Add mustard seeds. Let them pop up.
2. Then add cumin seeds, asafoetida powder, turmeric powder, cloves, red chilli powder.
4. Stuff the already made paste into the tomatoes by removing the pulp of tomatoes.
5. Then fry the tomatoes by adding it to the pan. Add salt, jaggery, and black pepper powder to it.
6. Cook this mixture for 10-15 minutes. After it becomes tender off the burner.

Note:
In this way stuffed tomato, capsicum, potatoes can be prepared. Gravy of onions, tomatoes can be added to this vegetable.

Mashed Potatoes

Ingredients:

Potatoes (medium sized)	3-4
Plain butter	1/4 cup
Black pepper powder	1/4 teaspoon
Salt to taste	

Benefits:

Easy to prepare.

Caution:

Persons suffering from constipation should not consume this recipe.

Method of preparation:

1. Boil the potatoes until they become soft and tender.
2. Then peel off the outer skin and mash the potatoes.
3. Add the other ingredients and blend the mixture. Serve hot.

Note for better taste:

Other spices such as coriander leaves, cumin seeds powder, asafoetida can also be added to relive flatulance.

Mushroom Bake

Ingredients:

Mushrooms	700 gms
Onions (medium sized)	1
Sesame oil	½ tablespoon
Plain flour	1 tablespoon
Sour cream	150 gms
Fresh wholemeal bread crumbs	20 gms
Low fat cheddar cheese	50 gms
Freshly ground black pepper	1 tablespoon
Brandy	1 tablespoon
Salt to taste	

Benefits:
Increases kapha and pitta. Low in cholesterol.

Method of preparation:
1. Wash the mushrooms.
2. Pat dry.
3. Roughly chop the onion.
4. Heat oil in a flameproof casserole with a tightly fitting lid.
5. Then add the chopped onion.
6. Cook gently for 5-7 minutes until lightly brown.
7. Pour in the brandy and heat for 5- 10 seconds, then standing well clear, ignite with a match.
8. When the brandy flames have subsided, stir in the flour & sour cream.
9. Heat gently for 5-6 minutes with constant stirring.
10. Don't allow boiling.
11. Add the mushrooms and remove the casserole from heat.
12. Add the salt and black pepper.
13. Then cover tightly with a lid.
14. Bake in the oven for 30 minutes until tender.
15. Remove from the oven & unlid.
16. Preheat the grill.
17. Mix the cheese (grated) with the breadcrumb & sprinkle over the mushrooms.
18. Brown under a hot grill.

Note for better taste:

Sweet- cured gammon rashers, about 75- 100 gms can be added while frying the onion. The dish can be garnished with chopped parsley. This is a German dish.

Non-Vegetarian

Chicken n' Spice

Ingredients:

Boneless chicken breast fillets	2
Garlic	3 cloves
Red chillies	2-3
Fresh ginger	20 gm
Coriander leaves	20 gm
Coriander seeds	1/2 teaspoon
Cumin seeds powder	1 teaspoon
Cardamom powder	1/4 teaspoon
Cinnamon powder	1/4 teaspoon
Turmeric powder	1/2 teaspoon
Clove powder	1 pinch
Nutmeg powder	1 pinch
Lemon juice	20 ml.
Pepper powder	1/4 teaspoon
Grated coconut	100 gm

Benefits:

Gives strength to the body; alleviates vata dosha.

Caution:

Not recommended in loss of appetite, haemorrhoids and obesity.

Method of preparation:

1. Mix all the spices and make it in a powdered form.
2. Place chicken, garlic, chillies, salt, in a bowl and mix it well.
3. Add the powders or spices to the chicken mixture and mix it well.
4. Cover and marinate it in refrigerator for 6 hours.
5. Add water and boil the mixture until chicken becomes tender.
6. Add lemon juice and mix it thoroughly. Now the Chicken N' Spice is ready to serve.

Note for better taste:

Garnish with coriander leaves.

Chicken Tikka

Ingredients:

Boned and skinned chicken breasts	4
Natural yoghurt	8 tablespoons
Garlic	1 clove
Tomato puree	1 tablespoon
Coriander	1-2 teaspoons
Turmeric powder	1 teaspoon
Chilli powder	1 teaspoon
Ginger paste	1 teaspoon
Cumin powder	2 teaspoons
Salt to taste	

Benefit:

Good for vata dosha. Increases pitta and reduces kapha.

Caution:

Wash and drain chicken properly or it will lead to some infection.

Method of preparation:

1. Lay the chicken breasts in a shallow dish.
2. Crush the garlic clove.
3. Mix the garlic with all the other ingredients thoroughly.
4. Pour the mixture all over the chicken and leave it to marinate for 2 hours.
5. Place the marinated chicken on a rack in the oven and position a backing tin underneath to catch any juices.
6. Cook for 25-30 minutes until the chicken is cooked.
7. Serve immediately.

Note for better taste:

This dish is served in Indian restaurants with rice.

Fish Puff

Ingredients:

White fish fillets	250 gm
Fresh ginger (finely chopped)	1 teaspoon
Green chillies (chopped)	1
Coriander leaves (finely chopped)	25 gm
Cumin seeds	1/2 teaspoon
Dried breadcrumbs	as required
Egg (lightly beaten)	1
Oil	2 tablespoons
Fresh lemon juice	1 teaspoon
Salt to taste	

Benefits:

Reduces vata dosha.

Caution:

Salt should be added with caution because fish are already preserved in salt.

Method of preparation:

1. Steam the boneless white fish fillets until just cooked.
2. Make pieces and place in a bowl.
3. Add all the spices and salt and mash with the fish flakes to combine.
4. Make lemon-size balls of the fish mixture.
5. Dip each ball in the egg mixture and roll in breadcrumbs to coat.
6. Heat the oil in a frying pan on a medium flame.
7. Fry the above balls in the oil until golden for 5 minutes.
8. Serve immediately.

Note for better taste:

The fish can be cooked in a microwave.
Other spices can be added according to the taste.

Indonesian Spicy Mutton

Ingredients:

Grated coconut	50 gm
Grated onions	200 gm
Red chillies	5
Boneless mutton	1/2 kg
Water	2 cups
Coriander seeds powder	4 teaspoon
Ginger (powder)	1 tablespoon
Cumin seeds powder	2 teaspoon
Curry leaves	5-6
Salt to taste	

Benefits:

Nourishes muscle tissue, reduces vata dosha.

Caution:

Individuals having hyperacidity should not consume this recipe.

Method of preparation:

1. Soak the red chillies in 1/2 cup of warm water for 15 minutes.
2. Make pieces of boneless mutton.
3. Make a paste of onions, chillies, and grated coconut.
4. Mix the paste and the mutton pieces thoroughly in a pressure pan.
5. Add all other ingredients and cover the pan with a lid.
6. Cook for 15 minutes on a low flame.
7. After the pressure is released remove the lid and stir well.

Note for better taste:

Any other meat can be used in place of mutton as per your taste.

Mince Meatballs

Ingredients:

Mutton mince/ beef mince	500 gms.
Pork or veal mince	150 gms.
Eggs	2
Chopped parsley	2 tablespoons
Grated nutmeg	1/4 teaspoon
Salt	1 tablespoon
Bread	5-6 slices
Milk	1 tablespoon
Oil	1 tablespoon

Benefits:

Good for vata. Increases pitta and kapha.

Caution:

Wash the mutton properly.

Method of preparation:

1. Beat 2 eggs till lightly mixed and keep aside.
2. Keep ready breadcrumbs softened in milk.
3. Combine all ingredients except the oil.
4. Shape the mixture into lemon size balls.
5. Sante the meat balls in batches in a frying pan till brown evenly.
6. Then set aside the balls.
7. Keep another frying pan on a low flame.
8. Add one tablespoon of oil to the pan.
9. Then ass meatballs and cover the pan.
10. Cook on a low flame for 15-20 minutes till tender.

Note for better taste:

Can be served with tomato sauce over pasta.
These meatballs can be stored in a rigid container and frozen for upto 3 months.

Pork Curry

Ingredients:

Red chillies	3
Ginger	5 gm
Garlic	4 cloves
Pepper powder	1/4 teaspoon
Coriander seeds & Turmeric powder	1/2 teaspoon each
Cumin seeds	1 teaspoon
Oil	1 tablespoon
Chopped onions	2
Chopped tomato	1
Boneless pork	1/2 kg
Green chillies	2
Chopped coriander & Chopped mint leaves	1 tablespoon each
Water	2-3 cups

Benefits:

It helps to gain weight and gives strength.

Caution:

Wash the meat properly.

Method of preparation:

1. Make a paste of ginger, garlic, pepper, cumin seeds, coriander seeds, red chillies by adding water.
2. Add oil to a pre heated pressure pan.
3. Fry the chopped onions till golden brown.
4. Add chopped tomatoes and stir well. Cook for five minutes.
5. Now add the above paste, meat and other ingredients.
6. Cook for ten minutes on a medium flame.
7. Add water and keep a lid on the pan and cook for fifteen minutes.
8. Allow the pressure to release on itself and then the recipe is ready to serve. Serve hot.

Note for better taste:

Vinegar can be used to make the paste of spices.

Sprouted Green Gram Paratha

Ingredients:

Wheat flour	200 gms
Sprouted green gram	60 gms
Water	200 ml
Coriander (chopped)	60 gms
Red chilli powder	1 teaspoon
Ghee	8 teaspoons
Turmeric powder	1 teaspoon
Lemon juice	2 teaspoons
Sesame oil	2 teaspoons
Salt to taste.	

Benefits:

Good for vata and pitta disorders.

Caution:

Too much of spices should not be added. Quantity of ghee should also be controlled or it will make the parathas heavy to digest.

Method of preparation:

1. Make soft dough of wheat flour by adding oil, salt and water.
2. Blend sprouted green gram, coriander, turmeric chilli powder and lemon juice.
3. Make small size balls of dough and blended mixture.
4. Make small circular rotis on flour board, stuff it with blended mixture.
5. Keep another circular roti on it.
6. Make round, thick paratha.
7. Roast it on non-stick fry pan for kapha constitution.
8. Or fry it on ghee on both sides for 10 minutes for vata constitution.

Note for better taste:

These parathas can be eaten with sauces.
In the same way, for stuffing the roti, crushed potatoes, cauliflower or leafy vegetables like fenugreek or spinach leaves.

Roti

Ingredients:

Wheat flour	500 gms
Sesame oil	3 teaspoons
Water	250 ml
Salt to taste.	

Benefits:

Balances tridoshas. Rotis can be digested easily because they are roasted.

Caution:

Before adding water make it lukewarm so that the dough becomes soft.

Method of preparation:

1. Take flour in a dish.
2. Add salt and oil to the flour.
3. Then add water and make soft dough by kneading.
4. Keep it aside for 15 minutes.
5. The dough can be made in a food processor also.
6. Then make lemon size balls of the dough.
7. Roll the ball on a floured board till it becomes thin and circular in shape from all sides.
8. Till you roll the balls heat an iron pan on a low flame.
9. Then roast the roti on the pan for 5-7 minutes from both the sides.

Note for better taste:

Rotis can be served with pure ghee or cheese or by applying jam. Another type of rotis called parathas can be prepared in the same way only by adding boiled potatoes or spinach or mixed vegetable to the wheat flour before making the dough.

RICE-DISHES

Rice and grains form the basis for healthy diet. Dozens of delicious sauces and curries can be added to make nutritious starters or simple but exciting main recipes.

Idli – Rice Cakes

Ingredients:

Rice	400 gms
Black gram	200 gms
Water as needed	
Salt to taste	

Benefits:

The idlies increases pitta. When there is vitamin deficiency this dish can be added to the regular diet, as this is a fermented product.

Caution:

The fermentation process should only be for 12 hrs and not more than that. Otherwise it will become sour to taste.

Method of preparation:

1. Soak the black gram and rice in water in the morning.
2. After 10- 12 hrs grind one by one, coarsely. Then mix both pastes.
3. Keep it for whole night to ferment.
4. In the morning add salt to taste and blend the mixture well.
5. Make it thin by adding little water.
6. Apply oil to the plates of idli maker so that while removing it can be easily removed & do not stick to the plates.
7. Add 2 teaspoons of mixture to the idli maker plates.
8. Cook it for 10 minutes in pressure cooker, without keeping pressure.
9. When idly gets properly cooked, off the burner. Check by putting the knife, it should not stick to the knife.

Note for better taste:

Idlis can be eaten with chutney or moong dal curry. It serves 4-5 persons and requires 30- 45 minutes.

Jeera Fried Rice

Ingredients:

Long grain rice	500 gms
Cumin seeds	2 tablespoons
Water	800 ml
Ghee/ Sesame oil	2 tablespoons
Salt to taste.	

Benefits:

Good for digestive fire (Jatharagni). Good for pitta & kapha.

Caution:

Don't add salt to rice while it is been boiled with water, as all essential nutrients will evaporate.

Method of preparation:

First plain rice is cooked by adding boiled water to rice in a pan.

1. Let it come to boil again.
2. Keep a lid on the pan.
3. Turn off the gas after the rice absorbs all the water.
4. Take another pan. Heat it. Add ghee/ oil to it.
5. Then add 2 tablespoons of the cumin seeds. Heat till brown. Now add already cooked rice in it.
6. Add salt in it and roast for atleast 5 minutes.
7. This serves 5 persons.

Khichari

Ingredients:

Long grain rice	500 gms
Green gram (split beans)	250 gms
Oil	2-3 tablespoons
Cumin seeds	1 tablespoons
Asafoetida powder	½ tablespoon
Turmeric powder	1 tablespoon
Red chilli powder	1 tablespoon
Mustard seeds	1 tablespoon
Grated coconut	50 gms
Coriander	50 gms
Water	800 ml
Salt to taste	

Benefits:
This recipe is used in Sansarjan krama, after doing Panchkar. Balances tridoshas. Increases digestive fires (agni).

Caution:
Add measured amount of water or it will lose its taste.

Method of preparation:
1. Wash and drain both rice and green grams.
2. Mix both.
3. Heat a non-stick pan.
4. Add oil in it. Keep the boiled water ready.
5. After heating the oil on low fire add cumin seeds, mustard seeds and asafoetida powder.
6. After the seeds pop up, add turmeric powder and then the mixture of rice & green gram dal to it.
7. Roast it for 5 minutes on low flame.
8. Add boiling water to the pan.
9. Cook for 10-15 minutes.
10. Add salt and chilli powder. Stir well.
11. Keep the lid & cook for 15 minutes on low flame till all the water is absorbed.
12. Garnish with grated coconut & chopped coriander leaves.

Note for better taste:
Sometimes dry fruits like pistachio, cashew nuts can also be added while cooking. But it is heavier to digest. Serve hot with soups or curry.

Rice

Ingredients:

Rice grains	100 gm
Water	500 ml

Benefits:

Rice is nutritious and reduces vata dosha. Without washing the grains of rice, it becomes heavy and increases kapha dosha.

Method of preparation:

1. Wash and drain the rice grains properly.
2. Then add water to it and cook for about 30 minutes by keeping lid over the pan.
3. As it becomes tender, off the burner.

Note for better taste:

Salt can be added according to taste. Earlier, rice grains can be roasted and then cooked by which rice becomes still lighter.

Spanish Rice

Ingredients:

Sesame oil	2 teaspoons
Medium onions	2
Garlic	1 clove
Ripe tomato & Pepper (red)	1 each
Skinned chicken thighs	4
Long-grain brown rice	250 gms
Ground turmeric	¼ teaspoon
Chicken stock/ water	550 ml
Paprika	1 teaspoon
Garlic sausage	50 gms
Frozen peas	100 gms
Unshelled prawns	150 gms

Salt and black pepper (ground) to taste.

Benefits:
Rice is high in fibre. Vitiates Pitta dosha due to spicy taste. Balances Vata & Kapha.

Caution:
Rice can be fried before cooking so it becomes light to digest.

Method of preparation:

1. Heat oil in a large frying pan.
2. Add chicken thighs and fry over a moderate heat till golden brown and remove from heat.
3. Chop the onions and crush the garlic and add to a pan. Cook gently for 5 minutes.
4. Dice tomato, de seed and dice the pepper.
5. Add tomato & pepper and cook for 2 minutes.
6. Add rice & turmeric, stir well and cook for 2 minutes.
7. Pour the stock or water into the pan & bring to boil.
8. Replace the chicken, cover & cook over a moderate heat for 15-20 minutes.
9. Then add garlic sausage & stir into the pan, add paprika & peas.
10. Cook for about 7-10 minutes without stirring, until all the liquid has been absorbed & the rice is cooked.
11. Peel the prawns keeping 4 prawns in their shells for garnish.
12. Add them to the pan and cook for 2-5 minutes.
13. Add salt & pepper to taste.
14. Whole process requires 1 hour.

Note for better taste: Served with a red wine punch gives a great taste.

DISEASE AND DIET

Introduction

Food is like a double-edged sword; it cures the disease as well as it may generate a disease if taken improperly. Your health entirely depends upon your daily diet. The diet should be chosen according to your agni, constitution, age, climate and ailment if any. Such a properly planned diet certainly helps to improve the health. Conversely improperly planned diet, wrong combinations may vitiate the health.

Most of the diseases we come across are the progeny of improper food and eating habits. Ayurveda understands disease as the imbalance of doshas and subsequently Panchamahabhutas. A planned diet for a particular disease is nothing but the supply of Panchamahabhutas required by the body e.g., in an over-nourished kind of a disease; tej, aakash & vayu dominant food should be supplied.

In the treatment, Ayurveda sees medicine and diet complimentary to each other. Usually medicines work according to their veerya (potency) and food according to the tastes primarily.

This module gives you basic idea to design your own diet pattern to make yourself more healthy, energetic and comfortable with your body. Here are some prescriptions and proscriptions according to the diseases.

Amavata (Rheumatoid Arthritis)

Aamavata is a chronic disorder, which affects the joints of the body. The precursor for this ailment is the 'aam', which is product of improper digestion. Indulgence in sexual activity, exercise etc. just after the meals; intake of food which is difficult for the digestive capacity to assimilate in the body may cause 'Aamavata'.

The symptoms observed are intense pain (like the scorpion bite), polyarthritis, improper digestion, loss of appetite, etc. Cardiac disorders, contractures in fingers of hands and feet etc. are the further manifestation of aamavata. Digestion of 'aam' and alleviation of vitiated vata are the two targets in the treatment of aamavata.

Proper dietetic pattern greatly benefits in relieving the symptoms. Consumption of heavy, sticky, very unctuous food certainly aggravates the disorder. In aamavata one has to consume food considering the appetite and quality of food primarily.
Aamavat (Rheumatoid arthritis)

Dos

English Name	Scientific Name
Fruits:	
Lime	*Citrus acida*
Lemon	*Citrus medica*
Mango steen	*Garcinia purpuria*
Papaya	*Carica papaya*
Vegetables:	
Agathi	*Aeschynomene grandiflora*
Hermaphrodite amarnath	*Amaranthus oleraceus*
Bathua leaves	*Chenopodium album*
Celery	*Apium graveolense*
Carrot leaves	*Daucus carota*
Coriander leaves	*Coriandrum sativum*
Curry leaves	*Murraya koenigii*
Drumstick leaves	*Moringa oleifera*
Indian sorrel	*Oxalis corniculata*
Red sorrel	*Rumex vesicaris*
Amala	*Emblica officinalis*
Bitter gourd	*Mormodica charantia*
Bottle gourd	*Langeria vulgaris*
Brinjal gourd	*Solanum melongena*
White variety of it should be consumed after roasting.	
Calabush cucumber	*Luffa aegyptiaca*

Ridge gourd/ Acute angled cucumber	*Luffa acuteangula*
Snake gourd	*Trichosanthes anguina*
<u>Roots & Tubers</u>:	
Beet root	*Beta vulgaris*
Carrot	*Daucus carota*
Onion	*Allium cepa*
Radish	*Raphenus sativus*
Yam	*Amorphophallus caupanulatus*
<u>Nuts</u>:	
Coconut	*Cocos nucifera*
<u>Oils</u>:	
Castor oil	*Ricinus communis*
One teaspoon full of castor oil can be taken with the dry ginger powder before meals.	
Safflower oil	*Carthamus tinctorius*
Sunflower oil	*Helianthus annus*
Less amount of oil should be consumed.	
<u>Cereals or Millets</u>:	
Bajra	*Pennisetum typhoideum*
Barley	*Hordeum vulgare*
Jowar	*Sorghum vulgare*
Maize, corn	*Zea mays*
Ragi	*Elucine coracana*
Rough chaft	*Achyranthus aspera*
<u>Pulses</u>:	
Green gram	*Phaseolus mungo*
Horse gram	*Dolichos biflorus*
Lentil dal	*Lens esculenta*
<u>Spices</u>:	
Asafoetida	*Ferula foetida*
Cardamom	*Elettaria cardamomur*
Chillies	*Capsicum aunum*
Cinamon	*Cinamomum zeylanicum*
Clove	*Eugenia caryophyllata*
Coriander	*Coriandrum sativum*
Cumin	*Cumimum cyminym*
Garlic	*Allium sativum*
Ginger	*Zingiber officinale*
Nutmeg	*Myristica fragrans*
Bishop's weed	*Carum roxburghianum*
Pepper	*Piper nigrum*
Fennel seeds	*Foeniculum vulgare*

Mustard seeds	*Brasica nigra*
Turmeric	*Curcuma longa*

Donts

English Name	Scientific Name
Fruits:	
Apple	*Pyrus malus*
Apricot	*Prunus armeniaca*
Banana	*Musa sapientum*
Bullocks heart	*Annona reticulata*
Cherries	*Prunus cerasus*
Custard apple	*Annona squamosa*
Dates	*Phoenix dactylifera*
Figs	*Ficus carica*
Figs are strongly contraindicated as they are one of the causative factors.	
Cluster fig	*Ficus glomerata*
Grapes	*Vitis vinifera*
Jack fruit	*Artocarpus integrifolia*
Jambul fruit	*Eugenia jambolana*
Orange	*Citrus reticulata*
Sweet orange	*Citrus aurantium*
Mango	*Mangifera indica*
Watermelon	*Citrullus vulgaris*
Palmyra palm	*Borassus flabelli formis*
Peach	*Prunus persica*
Pear	*Pyrus communis*
Pineapple	*Ananas sativus*
Pomegranate	*Punica granatum*
Raspberry	*Rubus lasiocarpus*
Strawberry	*Farigaria vesca*
Tomato	*Lycopersicum esculentum*
Wood apple	*Ferona elephantum*
Jujube	*Zizyphus jujuba*
Vegetables:	
Bengal gram leaves	*Cicer arietinum*
Brussel sprout	*Brassica olerasea*
Cabbage	*Brassica oleracea*
Fenugreek	*Trigonella foenum graeceum*
Garden cress/ Water cress leaves	*Lepidum sativum*
Mustard leaves	*Brasica nigra*

Spinach	*Spinacia olerecea*
Asparagus	*Asparagus officinalis*
Ash gourd	*Benincasa hispida*
Broad beans	*Faba vulgaris*
Double beans	*Faba vulgaris*
Cauliflower	*Brassica botrytis*
Cluster beans	*Cyamopsis psoralioides*
Cucumber	*Cucumis sativus*
French beans	*Phaseolus vulgaris*
Ladies finger/ Okra	*Hibiscus esculenthus*
Peas	*Pisum sativum*
Pumpkin	*Cucurbita maxima*
Soyabean	*Glycine soja*
<u>Roots and Tubers</u>:	
Potato	*Solanum tuberosum*
Sweet potato	*Ipomoea batatas*
<u>Nuts</u>:	
Almond	*Prunus amygdalus*
Cashew nut	*Anacardium occidentale*
Chest nut	*Aesculus hippocastanum*
Groundnut or peanut	*Arachis hypogaea*
Pistachio nut	*Pistacia vera*
Walnut	*Juglans regia*
Water chestnut	*Trapa bispinosa*
<u>Oils</u>:	
Gingelly seeds	*Sesamum indicum*
Groundnut oil	*Arachis hypogaea*
<u>Cereals or Millets</u>:	
Rice	*Oryza sativa*
Wheat	*Triticum sativum*
<u>Pulses</u>:	
Bengal gram or chick pea	*Cicer arietinum*
Black gram	*Phaseolus radiatus*
Cow gram	*Dolichos catiang*
Flat bean or Goa bean	*Dolichos lablab*
Red gram	*Cajanus indicus*
Horse gram	*Dolichos biflorus*
<u>Spices</u>:	
Tamarind	*Tamarindus indica*
<u>Miscellaneous</u>:	
Areca nut	*Areca catechu*

Betel leaves	*Piper betel*
Sago	*Sagus leavus*
Sugarcane	*Saccharum officinarum*
Yeast	*Cervisi actermeutum*
Hard cheese, butter	
Jaggery	
Sweet, sour and salty tastes in excess.	
Paneer	
Khoya	
Curds	
Though curds is rich in proteins and calories, it is abhishyandi. This property vitiates meda and mansa dhatu and aggravate the disease and hence is strongly contraindicated.	

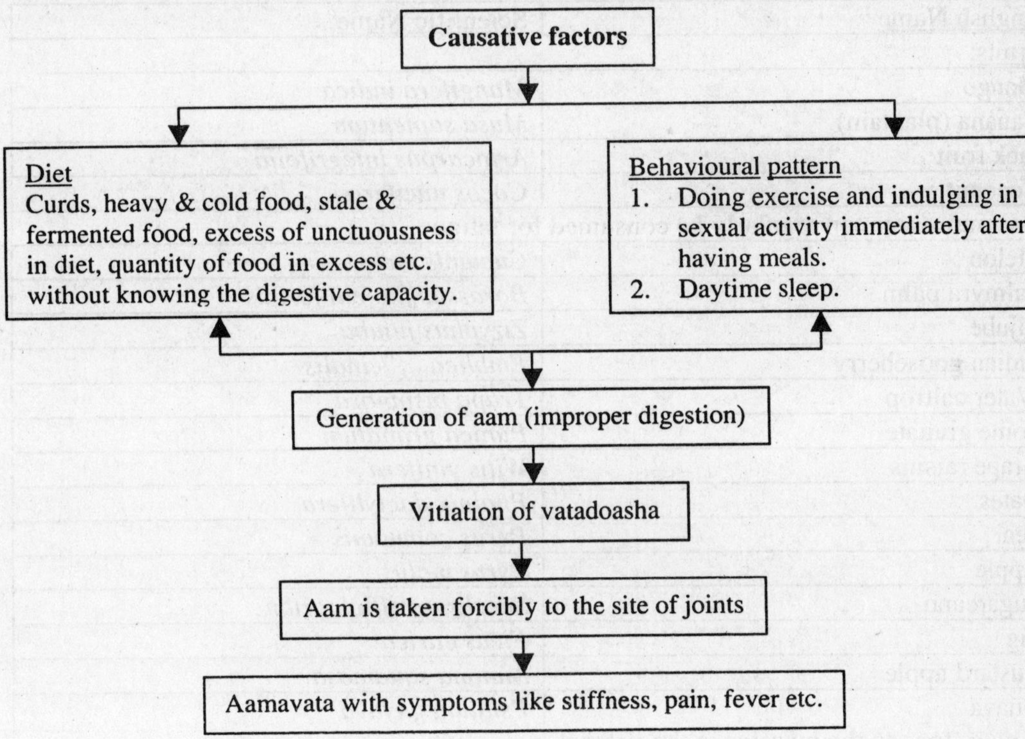

Aphrodisiac Diet

Good sexual relationship is one of the major aspects of a healthy married life. Healthy sexual intercourse is the most pleasuresome deed and the best remedy in stress management.

'Vatsyayan' the author of 'KAMASUTRA' the authority book on the subject, has praised the sexual deed as the experience of all the five senses at a time which relaxes the mind and the body as well. At the same time there causes the depletion of vital tissue of the body- 'SHUKRA'; and hence Ayurveda advocates Aphrodisiac treatment to all those who indulge themselves in sexual activity regularly. The diet pattern described here not only improves the quality and quantity of shukra, but also increases the vigour and desires upto some extent. This diet pattern is also beneficial for those who suffer from impotency of oligospermia.

Dos

English Name	Scientific Name
Fruits:	
Mango	*Mangifera indica*
Banana (plantain)	*Musa sapientum*
Jack fruit	*Artocarpus integrifolia*
Coconut	*Cocos nucifera*
Coconut water can regularly be consumed for fatigue.	
Melon	*Cucumis melo*
Palmyra palm	*Borassus flabelli formis*
Jujube	*Zizyphus jujuba*
Indian gooseberry	*Emblica officinalis*
Water caltrop	*Trapa bispinosa*
Pome granate	*Punica granatum*
Grape raisins	*Witis vinifera*
Dates	*Phoinix dactylifera*
Pear	*Pyrus communis*
Apple	*Pyrus malus*
Sugarcane	*Sacchrum officinarum*
Fig	*Ficus carica*
Custard apple	*Annona squamosa*
Guava It gives tone to the muscles in the vaginal path.	*Psidium guyava*
Papaya	*Carica papaya*
Vegetables:	

Cabbage	*Costus speciosus*
Okra or ladies finger	*Hibiscus esculenthus*
White goosefoot or Bathua leaves	*Chenopodium album*
Red malabar night shods	*Bassela rubra* *Bassela alba*
Chanchuki	*Carchorus acutangularis*
Ash gourd or white gourd melon	*Bennincasa hispida*
Sespadula	*Trichosanthus dioica*
Snake gourd	*Trichosanthus anguina*
Calabush cucumber	*Luffa pentandra*
Bottle gourd	*Langeria vulgaris*
Roots and Tubers:	
Beet root	*Beta vulgaris*
Carrot	*Daucus carota*
Onion	*Allium cepa*
Onion increases the sexual desire.	
Potato	*Solanum tuberosum*
Sweet potato	*Ipomoea batatas*
Nuts:	
Almond	*Prunus amygdalus*
Cashew nut	*Anacardium occidentale*
Walnut	*Juglans regia*
Pistachio nut	*Pistacia vera*
Ground nut	*Arachis hypogaea*
Oils:	
Groundnut oil	*Arachis hypogaea*
Coconut oil	*Cocos nucifera*
Cereal or Millets:	
Wheat	*Triticum sativum*
Rice	*Oryza sativa*
Pulses:	
Black gram	*Phaseolus radiatus*
Lentil	*Lens esculenta*
Spices:	
Cardamom	*Elettaria cardamomum*
Saffron	*Croci stigmata*
Nutmeg	*Myristica fragrans*
Nutmeg has the property of 'shukra stambhan' by which it relieves premature ejaculation.	
Dry ginger	*Zingiber officinalis*
Cinnamon	*Cinnamon cartex*

The back of the cinnamon should be used as it is aphrodisiac in nature. Whereas the leaves of the plant are anaphrodisiac and hence should not be used.	
Miscellaneous:	
Milk of buffalo, sheep, elephant Milk is a good aphrodisiac tonic. Milk with the spices and nuts can be regularly consumed. (Masala milk).	
Butter milk	
Curds Curds should be consumed with sugar or honey during daytime only. Preparation of curds like 'Rasala' can be regularly taken.	
Ghee (clarified butter) It should be consumed in regular diet.	
Meat Flesh of aquatic animals can be consumed as per the digestive capacity.	
Fishes from the rivers are aphrodisiac.	

Donts

English Name	Scientific Name
Fruits:	
Watermelon	*Citrullus vulgaris*
Wood apple	*Ferona elephantum*
Ebony	*Diospyros embryopteris*
Jambul fruit	*Eugenia jan bolana*
Stargoose berry	*Cicco dysticna*
Asiatic greevia	*Greevia asiatica*
Narrow leaved sepistun	*Cordia myza*
Vegetables:	
Pattashak	*Ipomea reprama*
Indian sorrel	*Oxalis corniculata*
Fenugreek	*Trigonella foenum graeceum*
Red sorrel	*Rumex vasicarius*
Cucumber	*Cucumis sativus*
Brinjal or eggplant	*Solanum melongena*
Ridge gourd or Acutangled cucumber	*Luffa acutengula*
Roots and Tubers:	
Yam	*Amorphopallus peniculatus*
Oils:	
Mustard oil	*Brasica nigra*
Safflower oil	*Carthamus tinctorius*
Sunflower oil	*Halianthus annus*

Cereals or Millets:	
Bajra	*Pennisetum typhoidicum*
Jowar	*Sorghum vulgare*
Barley	*Hordeum vulgare*
Chickling vetch	*Lathiyrus sativus*
Pulses:	
Cow gram	*Dolichos catiang*
Horse gram	*Dolichos biflorus*
Red gram	*Cajanus indicus*
Flat bean or Goa bean	*Dolichos lablab*
Bengal gram	*Cicer arietinum*
Nishpav	*Lebleb vulgaris*
Aconite leaved kidney bean	*Phaleolus aconitum*
Spices:	
Coriander seeds	*Coriandrum sativum*
These have the potential to alleviate the quality of all dhatus including shukra dhatu.	
Mustard seeds	*Brasica nigra*
Fennel seeds	*Foeniculum vulgare*
Miscellaneous:	
Areca nut	*Areca catechu*
Tobacco	
Alcohol	
Alcohol has all the attributes opposite to that of shukra dhatu and hence not recommended although it increases sexual desire.	

Constipation

This is a common symptom associated with indigestion, stomach upset etc. It can also be found as disease itself. Many a times chronic constipation leads to some anorectal disorders like haemorrhoids, fissure, rectal prolapse etc. Due to pressure induced at the time of defaecation, herniation of the intestine may be seen.

Some other major symptoms due to constipation include low backache, flatulance, angina, headache, muscular cramps etc. With the help of a specific diet pattern constipation can be treated upto some extent. The main key in the treatment of constipation is consumption of warm cooked food at regular meal timings (considering your hunger) and lukewarm water as far as possible.

Dos

English Name	Scientific Name
Fruits:	
Apple	*Pyrus malus*
Banana	*Musa sapientum*
Ripen banana is mild laxative.	
Fig	*Ficus carica*
Mango	*Mangifera indica*
Ripen mangoes help to relieve constipation	
Jack fruit	*Artocarpus integrifolia*
Lime	*Citrus acida*
Lime juice with warm water can be taken in the morning on empty stomach.	
Sweet orange	*Citrus cenesis*
Pomegranate	*Punica granatum*
Grape raisin	*Witis venifera*
This is a very good laxative which can be safely administered in infants also. Water with raisins soaked in it can be given to infants.	
Date	*Phoenix dactylifera*
Mulberry	*Morus indica*
Unripe mulberries are laxative.	
Kokam butter	*Garcinia purpuria*
This is a mild laxative; squash of it can be used in conditions like constipation in haemorrhoids, constipation with abdominal pain.	
Papaya	*Carica papaya*
Papaya tones up liver as well as spleen and relieve constipation. Papaya is strongly contraindicated in pregnant ladies.	
Vegetables:	
Bathua leaves (white goose foot)	*Chenopodium album*

It has a property to relieve constipation by increasing the digestive capacity.	
Red Malabar Night Shods	*Bassela rubra/ Bassela alba*
Being pruthvi and jala dominant it releives constipation.	
Marish	*Amaranthus tricalar*
It has two varieties red and white, of which red is mild laxative whereas white creates constipation.	
Hermaphrodite amaranath	*Amaranthus tenipolins*
Spinach	*Spinasia oleracea*
It relieves constipation but may create flatulence so it is advised to consume spinach with garlic, ginger, asafoetida etc.	
Kalashaka	*Phalugium tuberosum*
Purslane	*Portuiaca oleracea*
Out of two varieties, the bigger one is a laxative.	
Chanchuki	*Carchorus acutangularis*
Mustard leaves	*Brasica nigra*
Asparagus	*Asparagus officinalis*
Non Leafy Vegetables:	
Amla or Indian gooseberry	*Embelica officinale*
Bottle gourd	*Langeria vulgaris*
Bitter gourd	*Momordica charantia*
Sespadula	*Trichosanthus dioica*
Roots of this plant can be safely taken as a moderate laxative.	
Dindish (Tinde)	
Roots and Tubers:	
Potato	*Solanum tuberosum*
Onion	*Allium cepa*
Radish	*Raphanus sativus*
Beet root	*Beta vulgaris*
Nuts:	
Groundnut or Peanut	*Arachis hypogaea*
Cashew nut	*Anacardium occidentale*
Almond	*Prunus amygdalus*
Oils:	
Ground nut oil	*Arachis hypogaea*
Castor oil	*Ricinus communis*
Castor oil is a purgative. Dose can be adjusted depending upon bowel habits of an individual. One tablespoon of this oil can be taken with any foodstuff in the beginning of the meal. It oleates and brings back the unctuousness to the colons, and relieves constipation.	
Cereal or Millets:	

Barley	*Hordeum vulgare*
Wheat	*Triticum sativum*
Pulses:	
Black gram	*Phaseolus radiatus*
Horse gram	*Dolichos biflorus*
It is recommended in constipation with flatulance.	
Nishpav	*Lablab vulgaris*
Chinese dolicus	*Dolichos sinensis*
Spices:	
Asafoetida	*Ferula foetida*
It increases the digestive capacity and relieves flatulance, abdominal pain and discomfort.	
Cardamom	*Elettaria cardamomum*
Cumin seeds	*Cuminum cyminum*
Garlic	*Allium sativum*
Ginger	*Zinziber officinale*
A piece of wet ginger with rock salt should be consumed before meals daily.	
Fennel seeds	*Foeniculum vulgare*
Fennel seeds soaked in water can be consumed.	
Tamarind	*Tamarindus indica*
Tamarind squash can be consumed.	
Miscellaneous: .	
Freshly prepared buttermilk	
Cow's ghee	
Calorie conscious individuals restrict the intake of unctuous materials like ghee which inturn causes dryness of the colons.	

Donts

English Name	Scientific Name
Fruits:	
Unripe Banana	*Musa sapientum*
True custard apple of America or Sweetsop	*Annona reticulata*
Cluster fig	*Ficus glomerata*
Guava	*Psidium guyava*
Jambul fruit	*Eugenia jambolana*
Wood apple	*Ferona elephantum*
Asiatic greevia	*Greevia asiatica*
Zizyphus	*Zizyphus jujuba*
Jasmine flowered carissa	*Carissa congesta*

Watermelon	*Citrullus vulgaris*
Vegetables:	
Bengal gram leaves	*Cicer arietinum*
Mint	*Mentha arvenis*
Non Leafy Vegetables:	
Brinjal	*Solanum melongena*
Double beans	*Faba vulgaris*
Cluster beans	*Cyamopsis psoralioides*
Ladies finger or okra	*Hibiscus esculenthus*
Peas	*Pisum sativum*
Roots & Tubers:	
Sweet potato or Great leaved caledium	*Erum indicum*
Yam	*Dioscorea bulbifera*
Carrot	*Daucus carota*
Nuts:	
Pistachionut	*Pistacia vera*
Oil:	
Safflower oil	*Carthamus tinctorius*
Cereals or Millets:	
Bajra	*Pennisetum typhoidicum*
Jowar	*Sorghum vulgare*
Pulses:	
Bengal gram	*Cicer arietinum*
Flat bean or Goa bean	*Dolichos lablab*
Red gram	*Cajanus indicus*
Spices:	
Chillies	*Capsicum aunum*
Pepper	*Piper nigrum*
Turmeric	*Curcuma longa*
Miscellaneous:	
Areca nut	*Areca catechu*
Yeast	*Cervisi actermeutum*
Vinegar	
Red meat	

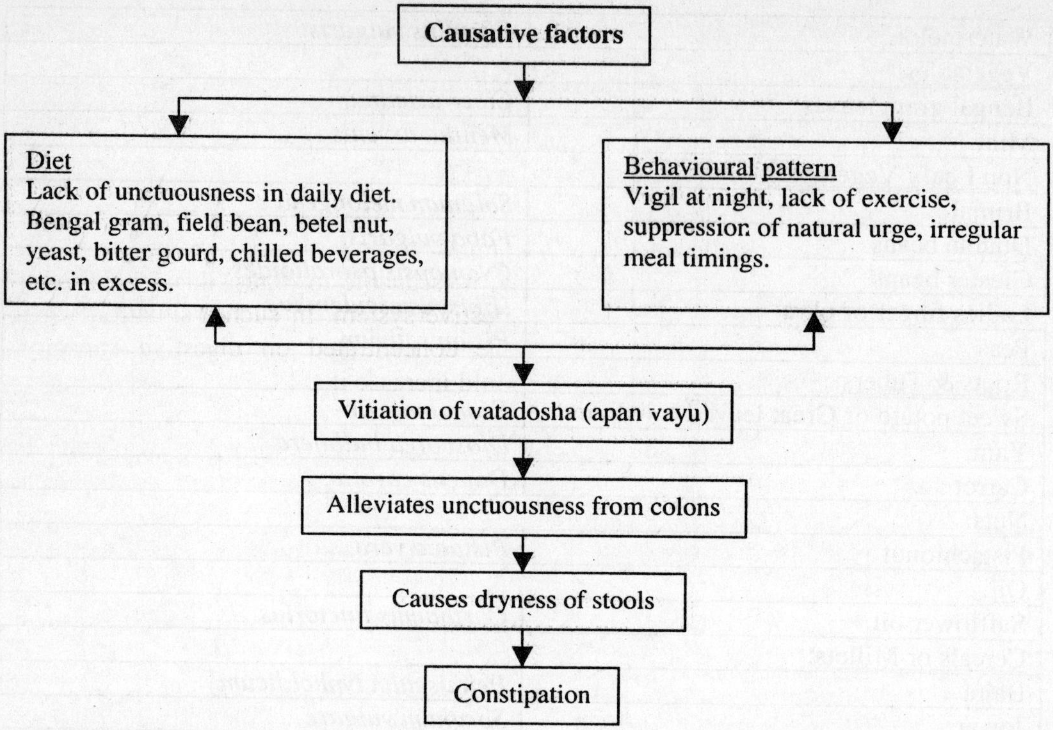
Causative factors
Diet
Lack of unctuousness in daily diet.
Bengal gram, field bean, betel nut,
yeast, bitter gourd, chilled beverages,
etc. in excess.
Behavioural pattern
Vigil at night, lack of exercise,
suppression of natural urge, irregular
meal timings.
Vitiation of vatadosha (apan vayu)
Alleviates unctuousness from colons
Causes dryness of stools
Constipation

Grahani (Irritable Bowel Syndrome)

This is a disorder of digestive system in which the strength of the digestive system, especially the small intestine is reduced uptó such an extent that functions like holding and absorption of food materials are hampered.

Consumption of heavy food when the digestive capacity is low may lead to Grahani. e.g. consumption of heavy meals, cheese, pork, milk products etc. during or just after diarrhoea. When the digestive capacity is low, it is unable to digest this much heavy food and in turn it becomes a load on the digestive system. In such a situation when digestive capacity is low, treatment is to be concentrated on digestive capacity. Supplying light food rather than heavy food should increase it.

Grahani presents symptoms like irregularity in the consistency of stools, (sometimes solid sometimes semisolid), increased frequency of defaecation, pain in abdomen, occurrence of food material in faeces, weight loss, hyperacidity, flatulance, mental irritability etc.

In treatment of this disorder, the digestive capacity should be increased primarily and simultaneously the strength of small intestine should also be increased.

As we know most of the disorders are the progeny of improper eating and eating habits, they can be cured or brought under control by following rules of eating correctly.

The food materials described should be cooked properly and consumed warm. Warm food stimulates the digestive capacity and helps to get it digested better.

Dos

English Name	Scientific Name
Fruits:	
Coconut	*Cocos nusifera*
Pomegranate	*Punica granatum*
Citron	*Citrus acida*
Squash of it with rock salt, black pepper can be consumed	
Lemon	*Citrus medica*
Sweet lemon	*Citrus aurantium*
Kokam butter	*Garcinia purpuria*
Asiatic greevia	*Greevia asiatica*
Water caltrop	*Trapa bispinosa*
Wood apple This should be consumed unripen.	*Ferona elephantum*

Dates	*Phoenix Montana* or *Phoenix sylvestris*
Dates should be consumed when the appetite is increased.	
Water melon	*Citrus vulgaris*
Papaya	*Carica papaya*
Papaya should never be consumed in pregnancy.	
Lime	*Citrus acida*
Vegetables:	
Cabbage	*Brassica oleracea*
Purslane	*Portuiaca oleracea*
The smaller variety is recommeded in IBS.	
Siriyari	*Blepharis edulis*
Brinjal	*Solanum melongena*
White variety of brinjals should be consumed.	
Drumstick leaves	*Morringa oleifera*
Cucumber	*Cucumis sativus*
Sespadula	*Trichosanthis cucumerina*
Acuteangled cucumber	*Luffa acuteangula*
Snake gourd	*Trichosanthis anguina*
Lettuce	*Lactuca scariola*
Bitter gourd	*Momordica charantia*
Bitter gourd increases digestive capacity and helps digestion. However in excess it acts as a mild laxative.	
Asparagus	*Asparagus officinalis*
Cauliflower	*Brassica botrytis*
Mint	*Mentha arvenis*
Indian sorrel	*Oxalis corniculata*
Coriander	*Coriandrum sativum*
Carrot leaves	*Daucus carota*
Celery leaves	*Apium graveolense*
Roots & Tubers:	
Yam	*Amorphopallus peniculatus*
Radish	*Raphanus sativus*
Carrot	*Daucus carota*
Beet root	*Beta vulgaris*
Onion	*Allium cepa*
Roasted onions can be consumed	
Oils and Ghees:	
Sunflower oil	*Halianthus annus*
Safflower oil	*Carthamus tinctorius*

Less amount of oil should be used for cooking.	
Cow's ghee Should be consumed in daily diet.	*Clarified butter*
Cereal or Millets:	
Barley	*Hordeum vulgare*
Jawar	*Sorghum vulgare*
Maize, corn	*Zea mays*
Ragi	*Elucine coracana*
Rice	*Oryza sativa*
All grains should be roasted before preparation	
Pulses:	
Green gram	*Phaseolus mungo*
Aconite leaved kidney bean	*Phaseolus aconitum*
Lentil	*Lens esculenta*
Spices:	
Asafoetida	*Ferula foetida*
Releives abdominal pain, flatulance; 125 mg. should be consumed with cow's ghee.	
Cinnamon	*Cinnamomum zeylanica*
Folia malabathy	*Cinnamomum tamala*
Saffron	*Croci stigmata*
Clove	*Caropyhyllus aromaticus*
Cardamom	*Elettaria cardamomum*
Nutmeg Beneficial in diarrhoea.	*Myristica fagrans*
Turmeric	*Curcuma longa*
Cumin seeds	*Cumimum cyminym*
Garlic	*Allium sativum*
Ginger Dry ginger is beneficial in IBS	*Zinziber officinale*
Pepper	*Piper nigrum*
Coriander	*Coriandrum sativum*
Mustard seeds	*Brasica nigra*
Fennel seeds	*Foeniculum vulgare*
Miscellaneous:	
Buttermilk.	
Buttermilk with pepper powder, rock salt, ginger, etc. is the best thing for IBS. It increases appetite as well as gives strength to the intestine.	
Plain butter	
Betel leaves	*Piper betel*
Flesh of pigeon	

Donts

English Name	Scientific Name
Fruits:	
Banana	*Musa sapientum*
Cashew fruit	*Anacardium occidentale*
Mango	*Mangifera indica*
Jack fruit	*Artocarpus integrifolia*
Date	*Phoenix dactylifera*
Apple	*Pyrus malus*
Mulberries	*Morus indica*
Sugar cane	*Saccharum officinarum*
Fig	*Ficus carica*
Bokhera plum	*Cherry plum*
Grapes	*Vitis vinifera*
Palmyra palm	*Borassus flabelli formis*
Pineapple	*Ananas sativus*
Strawberry	*Farigaria vesca*
Raspberry	*Rubus lasiocarpus*
Tomato	*Lycopersicum esculentum*
Jujube	*Zyzyphus Jujube*
Vegetables:	
Hermaphrodite amaranth	*Amaranthus tenipolins*
Bathua leaves	*Chenopodium album*
Bengalgram leaves	*Cicer oleracea*
Fenugreek leaves	*Trigonella foenum graeceum*
Dill leaves	*Peucedanum graveolens*
Red sorrel (field sorrel)	*Hibiscus sabdariffa*
Spinach	*Spinacia olerecea*
Ash gourd	*Benincasa hispida*
Broad beans	*Faba vulgaris*
Double beans	*Faba vulgaris*
Cluster beans	*Cyamopsis psoralioides*
French beans	*Phaseolus vulgaris*
Ladies finger/ okra	*Hibiscus esculenthus*
Peas	*Pisum sativum*
Pumpkin	*Cucurbita maxima*
Soyabean	*Glycine soja*
Roots and tubers:	
Potato	*Solanum tuberosum*
Sweet potato	*Ipomoea batatas*
Nuts and oil seeds:	

Almonds	*Prunus amygdalus*
Cashew nut	*Anacardium occidentale*
Pistachio nut	*Pistacia vera*
Walnut	*Juglans regia*
Water chestnut	*Trapa bispinosa*
Castor seeds	*Ricinus communis*
Cereal or Millets:	
Oats	*Avena sativa*
Wheat	*Triticum sativum*
Pulses:	
Bengal gram or chick pea	*Cicer arietinum*
Black gram	*Phaseolus radiatus*
Horse gram	*Dolichos biflorus*
Pigeon pea	*Cajanus indicus*
Spices:	
Chillies	*Capsicum aunum*
Tamarind	*Tamarindus indica*
Miscellaneous:	
Hard cheese	
Buffalo's milk	
Tobacco	
Areca nut	*Areca catechu*
Yeast	*Cervisi actermeutum*
Sago	*Sagus leavus*
Flesh of animals; fish etc.	

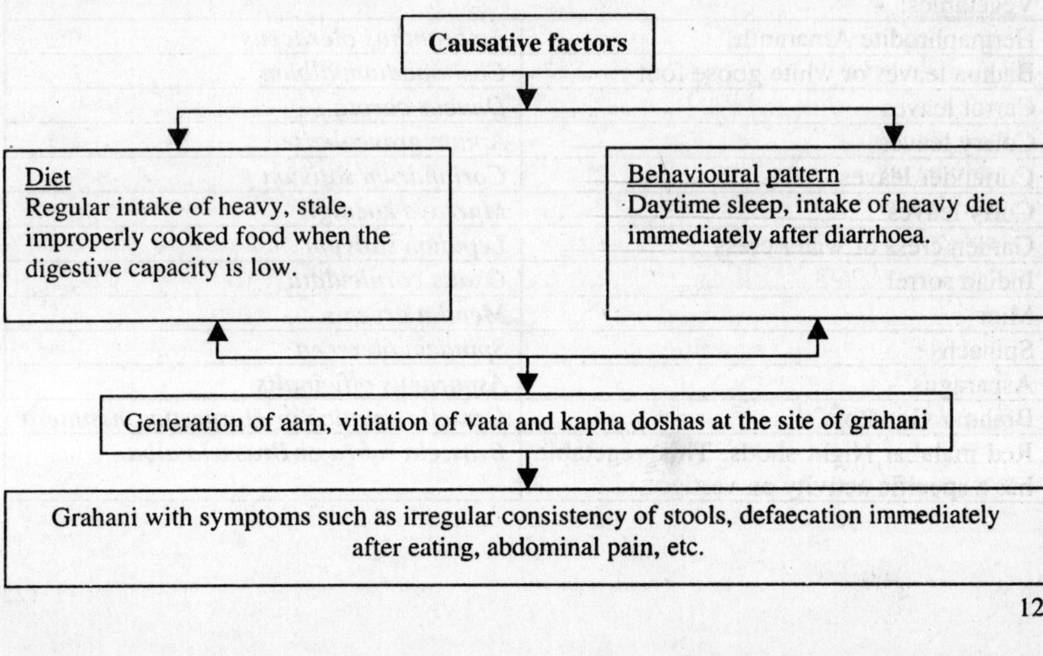

Hyperacidity

This is the commonest disease usually associated with symptoms such as heart burn, sour belch, giddiness, nausea etc. The foodstuffs antagonistic to eaçh other; rotten, toxic, pungent and sour foodstuffs; spicy; heavy; hot, unctuous/ dry-in excess, intake of water in excess, rice flakes, partly fermented alcohol, ragi, sour buttermilk, dry vegetables etc. should not be consumed. Frequent eating, fasting, sleeping after meals, consumption of stale food etc. should also be avoided. All these factors vitiate pitta dosha, which inturn leads to Amla pitta (Hyperacidity).

Dos

English Name	Scientific Name
Fruits	
Apple	*Pyrus malus*
Banana	*Musa sapientum*
Dates	*Phoenix dactylifera*
Figs	*Ficus carica*
Grape raisins	*Witis vinifera*
Jambul fruit	*Eugenia jambolana*
Coconut	*Cocus nucifera*
Sweet orange	*Citrus aurantium*
Mango	*Mangifera indica*
Mango pulp should be consumed with a pinch of pepper powder and ghee in it.	
Pomegranate	*Punica granatum*
Wood apple	*Ferona elphantum*
Kokam butter	*Garcinia purpuria*
Vegetables:	
Hermaphrodite Amaranth	*Amaranthus oleraceus*
Bathua leaves or white goose foot	*Chenopodium album*
Carrot leaves	*Daucus carota*
Celery leaves	*Apium graveolense*
Coriander leaves	*Coriandrum sativum*
Curry leaves	*Murraya koenigii*
Garden cress or water cress	*Lepidum sativum*
Indian sorrel	*Oxalis corniculata*
Mint	*Mentha arvenis*
Spinach	*Spinacia olerecea*
Asparagus	*Asparagus officinalis*
Brahmi/ Gotukola	*Centella asiatica or Herpestics monniera*
Red malabar Night shods. This vegetable has a specific activity on vertigo.	*Brassela rubra* or *Brassela alba*

Non Leafy Vegetables:	
Amla or Indian gooseberry	*Emblica officinalis*
White pumpkin	*Benincasa hispida*
Bitter gourd	*Mormodica charantia*
Bottle gourd	*Langeria vulgaris*
Cabbage	*Costus speciosus* or *Brassica oleracea*
Pumpkin	*Cucurbita maxima*
Ridge gourd	*Luffa acutangula*
Roots & Tubers:	
Beet root	*Beta vulgaris*
Carrot	*Daucus carota*
Sweet potato	*Ipomoea batatas*
Great leaved caledium	*Erum indicum*
Pulses:	
Green gram	*Phaseolus mungo*
Bengal gram	*Cicer arietinum*
Lentil	*Lens esculenta*
Black gram	*Phaseolus radiatus*
Bengal gram and Lentils in excess may create flatulance and hence should not be consumed frequently.	
Spices:	
Garlic	*Allium sativum*
Garlic soaked in sour buttermilk for 4 hours can be safely consumed in hyperacidity which otherwise is not recommended.	
Coriander	*Coriandrum sativum*
Cumin seeds	*Cumimum cyminym*
Cumin seeds can be consumed in hyperacidity with flatulance.	
Dry Ginger	*Zinziber officinale*
Nuts:	
Coconut	*Cocus nucifera*
Oils:	
Sunflower oil	*Hallianthus annus*
Safflower oil	*Carthamus tinctorius*
Coconut oil	*Cocus nucifera*
Cereal or Millets:	
Barley	*Hordeum vulgare*
Jowar	*Sorghum vulgare*
Wheat	*Triticum sativum*
Ragi	*Elucine coracana*
Spices:	
Saffron	*Croci stigmata*

Clove	*Caryophylus aromaticus*
Nutmeg	*Myristica fragrans*
Nutmeg is beneficial in the vomiting symptom of hyperacidity and 125 mg. of it can be taken with honey.	
Turmeric	*Curcuma longa*
<u>Miscellaneous</u>:	
Cow's milk Preheated cow's milk is a good antacid.	
Buttermilk	
Clarified butter	
Plain butter	

Donts

<u>English Name</u>	<u>Scientific Name</u>
<u>Fruits</u>	
Bokhera plum	*Cherry plum*
Jack fruit	*Artocarpus integrifolia*
Watermelon	*Citrullus vulgaris*
Cherry	*Prunus cerasus*
Cashew fruit	*Anacardium occidentale*
Lime	*Citrus acida*
Grape fruit	*Citrum parodisi*
Orange	*Citrus reticulata*
Tomato	*Lycopersicum esculentum*
Pineapple	*Ananas sativus*
Plum	*Prunus domistica americana*
Any tinned fruit juice with the preservatives in it, is strongly contraindicated. Similarly any unripe fruit with sour taste should not be consumed.	
<u>Vegetables</u>:	
Fenugreek	*Trigonella foenum graeceum*
Dill leaves	*Peucedanum graveolens*
Red sorrel or Field sorrel	*Hibiscus sabdariffa*
Drum stick leaves	*Moringa oleifera*
Mustard leaves	*Brasica nigra*
Brinjal gourd	*Solanum melongena*
Cluster bean	*Cyamopsis psoralioides*
<u>Nuts</u>:	
Peanut or groundnut	*Arachis hypogaea*
<u>Oil</u>:	
Mustard oil	*Brasica nigra*

Sesame oil	*Sesasum indicum*
Any oil in excess	
<u>Cereal or Millets</u>:	
Bajra	*Pennisetum typhoidicum*
<u>Pulses</u>:	
Horse gram	*Dolichos biflorus*
Cow gram or Chinese Dolicas	*Dolichos catiang*
Red gram	*Cajanus indicus*
<u>Spices</u>:	
Asafoetida	*Ferula foetida*
Cardamom	*Elettaria cardamomum*
Chilli	*Capsicum aunum*
Cinnamon	*Cinamomum zeylanicum*
Pepper Pepper powder should not be consumed in excess.	*Piper nigrum*
Tamarind	*Tamarindus indica*
Mustard seeds	*Brasica nigra*
<u>Miscellaneous</u>:	
Betel leaves	*Piper betel*
Yeast	*Cervisi actermeutum*
Paneer	
Vinegar	
Fish and flesh of aquatic animals	
Curds	
Sour buttermilk	

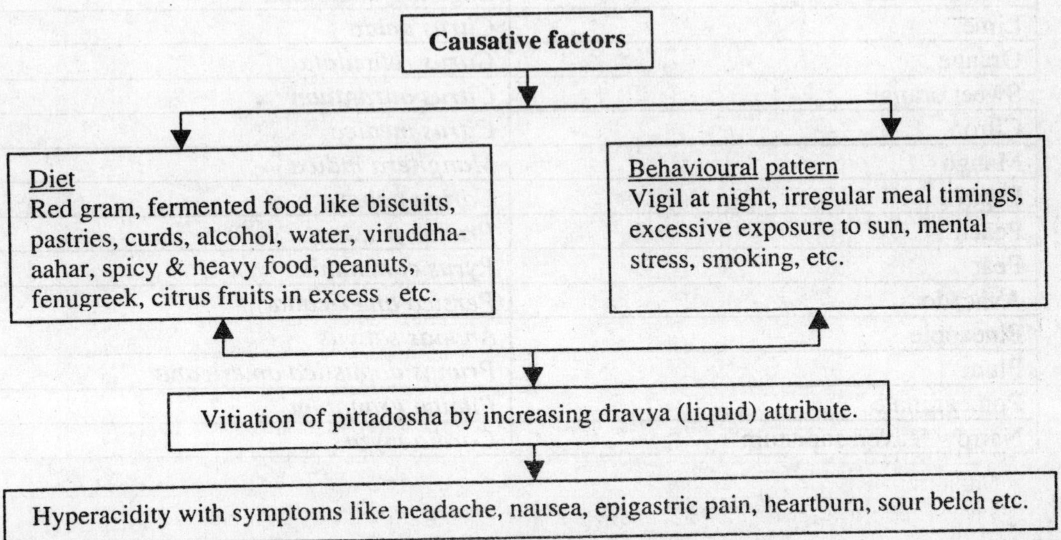

Kushtha (Skin Disorder)

Almost all the skin disorders are due to wrong combinations of food , contraindicated food and suppression of natural urges. These wrong combinations include consumption of fruits with milk; radish with milk etc. In today's world of 'calorie consciousness', milk shakes of fruits are one of the best nutrients, but Ayurveda strongly proscripts such type of diet. Although pathogenesis of skin disorders is a long process, regular intake of such food items vitiate rasa, rakta and mansa dhatu gradually create various skin disorders.

Vomiting is a natural urge of the body which if suppressed may lead to a skin disease. In the same way, experiencing two extreme conditions of temperature simultaneously may also act as a causative factor to the skin disease. Cold water bath just after steam or sauna is very common behaviour seen everywhere. Such things create imbalance in doshas. The diet pattern described here, helps to bring back doshas to the normalcy.

Dos

English Name	Scientific Name
Fruits:	
Apple	*Pyrus malus*
Banana	*Musa sapientum*
Cashew fruit	*Anacardium occidentale*
Cherry	*Prunus cerasus*
Dates	*Phoenix dactylifera*
Fig	*Ficus carica*
Cluster fig	*Ficus glomerata*
Grapes	*Vitis vinifera*
Jack fruit	*Artocarpus integrifolia*
Jambul fruit	*Eugenia jambolana*
Lime	*Citrus acida*
Orange	*Citrus reticulata*
Sweet orange	*Citrus aurantium*
Citron	*Citrus medica*
Mango	*Mangifera indica*
Papaya	*Carica papaya*
Peach	*Prunus persica*
Pear	*Pyrus communis*
Avacado	*Persica americana*
Pineapple	*Ananas sativus*
Plum	*Prunus domistica americana*
Pomegranate	*Punica granatum*
Narrow leaved sapistum	*Cordia myza*

Wood apple	*Ferona elephantum*
Jujube	*Zizyphus jujuba*
Spondias minute	*Spondias mangifera*
Ebony	*Diospiros embryopteris*
Stargoose berry	*Phylanthus distinchus*
Obtuse leaved mimusobs	*Mimusobs hexendra*
Water caltrop	*Trapa bispinosa*
Releives burning sensation	
Elloopa tree	*Basia longifolia*
Asiatic greevia	*Greevia asiatica*
Mustard tree of scripture	*Salvadora parsica*
Kokam butter	*Garcinia purpuria*
Vegetables:	
Bathua leaves white goose foot	*Chenopodium album*
Spinach	*Spinasia oleracea*
Mint	*Mentha sylvestris*
Coriander leaves	*Coriandrum sativum*
Kessoor	*Scripus kessoor*
Releives burning sensation	
Hermaphrodite amaranth	*Amaranthus tenipolins*
Kalashak	*Phalugium tuberosum*
Releives oedema	
Indian sorrel	*Oxalis corniculata*
Siriyari	*Blepharis edulis*
Round podded cassia	*Cassia sophera*
Cabbage	*Brasica oleraseb capita*
Carrot leaves	*Daucus carota*
Celery leaves	*Apium graveolens*
Curry leaves	*Murraya koenigii*
Drumstick leaves	*Moringa olefera*
Small carltrops	*Boerrhavia diffusa*
Ash gourd	*Benincasa hispida*
Bitter gourd	*Momordica charantia*
Bottle gourd	*Langeria vulgaris*
Okra or Ladies finger	*Hibscus esculenthus*
French beans	*Phaseolus vulgaris*
Snake gourd	*Trichosanthes anguina*
Ridge gourd	*Luffa acutengula*
Roots and Tubers:	
Beet root	*Beta vulgaris*
Carrot	*Daucas carota*

Onion	*Allium cepa*
Potato	*Solanum tuberosum*
Radish	*Raphanus sativus*
Nuts:	
Coconut	*Cocus nucifera*
Oils:	
Safflower oil	*Carthamus tinctorius*
Sunflower oil	*Helianthus annus*
Olive oil	*Olea europoea*
Castor oil	*Ricinus communis*
Cereals or Millets:	
Bajra	*Pennisetum typhoidicum*
Barley	*Hordeum vulgare*
Jowar	*Sorghum vulgare*
Maize	*Zea mays*
Ragi	*Elucine coracana*
Wheat	*Triticum sativum*
Pulses:	
Green gram	*Phaseolus mungo*
Lentil dal	*Lens esculenta*
Black gram	*Phaseolus radiatus*
Spices:	
Asafoetida	*Feruls foetida*
Cardamom	*Elettaria cardamomum*
Cinnamon	*Cinamomum zeylanicum*
Clove	*Eugenia caryophyllata*
Coriander seeds	*Coriandrum sativum*
Cumin seeds	*Cuminum cyminum*
Garlic	*Allium sativum*
Ginger	*Zingiber officinale*
Nutmeg	*Myristica fragrans*
Bishop's weeds	*Carum roxburghianum*
Pepper	*Piper nigrum*
Fennel seeds	*Foeniculum vulgare*
Turmeric	*Curcuma longa*
Tamarind	*Tamarindus indica*
Saffron	*Croci stigmata*
Miscellaneous:	
Unsalted butter	
Ghee made of cow's milk	
Camphor mixed with water can be consumed.	

Donts

English Name	Scientific Name
Fruits:	
Custard apple	*Annona squamosa*
Guava	*Psidium guyava*
Palmyra palm	*Borasus flabelli formis*
Unripe mango	*Mangifera indica*
Strawberry	*Farigaria vesca*
Raspberry	*Rubus lasiocarpus*
Mulberry	*Morus indica*
Tomato	*Lycopersicum esculentum*
Melon	*Cucumis melo*
Lakooch	*Artocarpus lacoochaii*
Watermelon	*Citrullus vulgaris*
Jasmine flowered carissa	*Carissa corandal*
Vegetables:	
Bengal gram leaves	*Cicer arietinum*
Mustard leaves	*Brasica nigra*
Brinjal	*Solanum melongena*
Broad beans	*Faba vulgaris*
Double beans	*Faba vulgaris*
Calabash cucumber	*Luffa aegyptiaca*
Cluster beans	*Cyamopsis psoralioides*
Cucumber	*Cucumis sativus*
Peas	*Pisum sativum*
Soyabean	*Glycine soja*
Roots and Tubers:	
Yam	*Dioscorea bulbifera*
Nuts:	
Groundnut	*Arachis hypogaea*
Cashew nut	*Anacardium occidentale*
Chest nut	*Aesculus hippocastanum*
Pistachio nut	*Pistacia vera*
Walnut	*Juglans regia*
Water chestnut	*Trapa bispinosa*
Oils:	
Sesame oil	*Sesamum indicum*
Cotton seed oil	*Gossypium herbaceum*
Pulses:	
Horse gram	*Dolichos biflorus*
Bengal gram	*Cicer arietinum*

Red gram	*Cajanus indicus*
Flat bean or Goa bean	*Dolichos lablab*
Miscellaneous:	
Tobacco	
Betel nut	
Sago	*Sagus leavus*
Vinegar	
Yeast	*Cervisi actermeutum*
Mushrooms	
Alcohol	
Curds	
Fruit milkshakes	
Hard cheese	
Milk with salt	
Fish and milk	
Meat with curds	

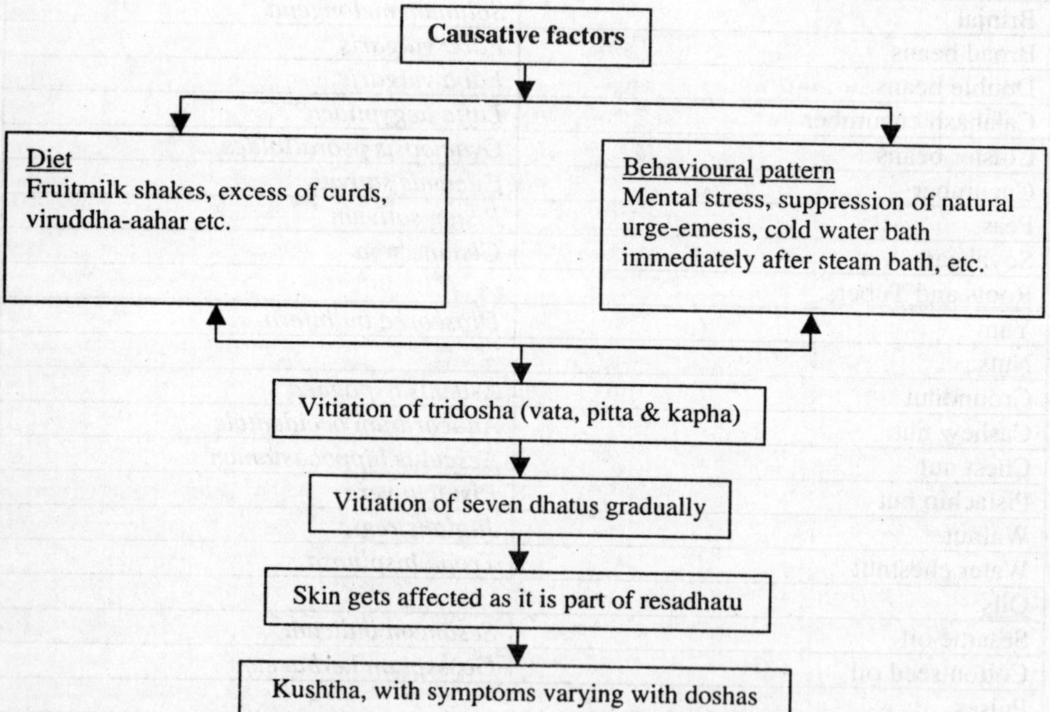

Nidranaash (Insomnia)

Good amount of sleep is very necessary for the health of every individual. Vigil at night vitiates vata dosha by depleting unctuousness and may generate various disorders. Daytime sleep increases unctuiousness which in turn vitiates kapha dosha. Persons suffering from disorders of throat and intoxication are not advised to sleep, until the ailment is cured.

Insomnia may give rise to symptoms such as body ache, heaviness in head, yawning, difficulty in grasping the knowledge, indigestion and disorders of vata dosha. The ill effects caused by vigilance can be corrected by taking a nap for half the time of vigilance before intake of food.

Quality and quantity wise proper sleep tries to balance the level of doshas and relaxes the sense organs and mind.

Dos

English Name	Scientific Name
Fruits:	
Apple	*Pyrus malus*
Banana	*Musa sapientum*
True custard apple of America or Sweetsop	*Annona reticulata*
Cashew fruit	*Anacardium occidentale*
Cherry	*Prunus cerasus*
Custard apple	*Annona squamosa*
Dates	*Phoenix dactylifera*
Fig	*Ficus carica*
Grapes	*Vitis vinifera*
Jack fruit (ripen)	*Artocarpus integrifolia*
Lime	*Citrus acida*
Orange	*Citrus reticulata*
Mango	*Mangifera indica*
Palmyra palm	*Borasus flabelliformis*
Melon	*Cucumis melo*
Pomegranate	*Punica granatum*
Poison nut	*Strychnos nuxvomica*
Jasmine flowered carissa	*Carissa corandal*
Elloopa tree	*Bassia longifolia*
Vegetables:	
Red malabar night shods	*Bassela alba* or *Bessela rubra*

Cabbage	*Brasica oleraseb capita*
Garden cress or water cress	*Lepidum sativum*
Gotukola	*Centella asiatica*
White pumpkin	*Benincasa hispida*
Pumpkin	*Cucurbita maxima*
Bottle gourd	*Langeria vulgaris*
Soybean	*Glycine soja*
Roots and Tubers:	
Potato	*Solanum tuberosum*
Sweet potato	*Ipomoea batatas*
Yam	*Dioscorea bulbifera*
Nuts:	
Walnut	*Juglans regia*
Cashew nut	*Anacardium occidentale*
Coconut	*Cocus nucifera*
Head massage with coconut oil gives sound sleep.	
Oils:	
Groundnut oil	*Hypogaca arachic*
Olive oil	*Olea europoea*
Cereals or Millets:	
Rice	*Oryza sativa*
Ragi	*Elucine coracana*
Wheat	*Triticum sativum*
Pulses:	
Nutmeg	*Myristica fragrans*
Bishop's weeds	*Carum roxburghianum*
Black gram	*Phaseolus radiatus*
Poppy seeds	*Papaver somniferum*
Miscellaneous:	
Sago	*Sagus leavus*
Buffalo's milk It should be consumed before going to bed.	
Red meat	
Wines	

Donts

English Name	Scientific Name
Fruits:	
Guava	*Psidium guyava*

Apricot	*Prunus armeniaca*
Jambul fruit	*Eugenia jambolana*
Cluster fig	*Ficus glomerata*
Lakooch	*Artocarpus lacoochaii*
Tomato	*Lycopersicum esculentum*
Watermelon	*Citrullus vulgaris*
Papaya	*Carica papaya*
Wood apple	*Ferona elephantum*
Vegetables:	
Brinjal	*Solanum melongena*
Bitter gourd	*Mormodica charantia*
Roots and Tubers:	
Onion	*Allium cepa*
Radisl.	*Raphanus sativus*
Spices:	
Black pepper	*Piper nigrum*
Chillies	*Capsicum aunum*
Ginger	*Zinziber officinale*
Asafoetida	*Ferula foetida*
Cardamom	*Elettaria cardamomum*
cinamon	*Cinnamomum zeylanicum*
Cumin	*Cuminum cyminum*
Miscellaneous:	
Areca nut	*Areca catechu*
Betel leaves	*Piper betel*

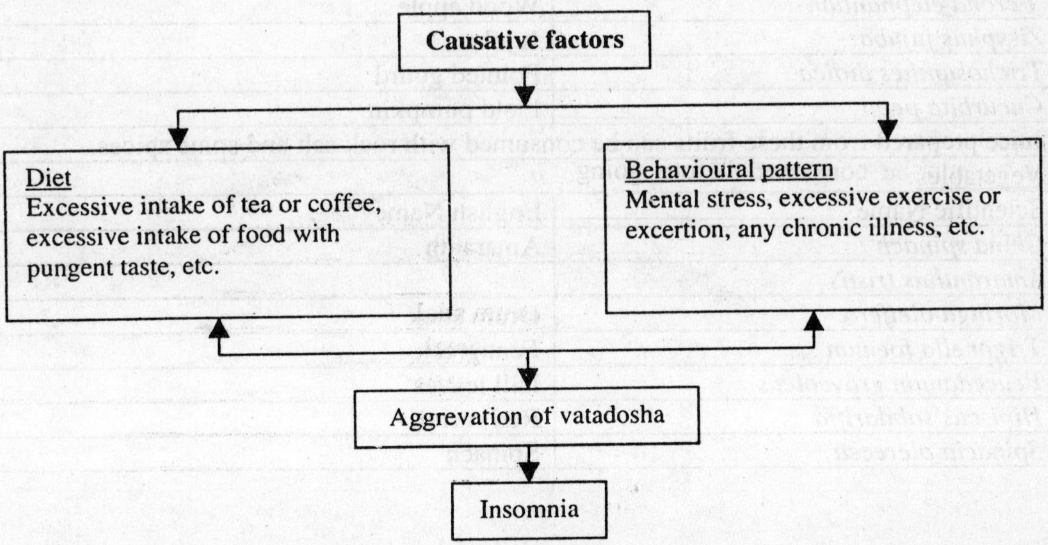

Obesity

Dietetic Regimen:

Obesity is more a tendency than a disease; commonly found in the affluent class all over the World.

There is a significant number of people who have many serious, life threatening illnesses brought out by obesity like cardiac disorders, hypertension, stroke, diabetes and some types of cancer. Diet is a major factor in maintaining weight of an individual. Ayurveda emphasises on the quality of the food more than the quantity. The diet based on calorie count i.e., severely restricting the intake of food doesn't help to lose weight, particularly over a longer period, because usually the lost weight is regained after certain period of time. And such "yo-yo" kind of therapy is more hazardous than being overweight all the time. The diet pattern we recommend helps the body to accomplish proper heath by loosing the weight.

Dos

Scientific Name	English Name
Fruits:	
Psidium guyava	Guava
Eugenia jambolana	Jambul fruit
Ficus glomerata	Cluster fig
Citrus Fruits:	
Citrus acida	Lime
Citrus reticulata	Orange
Citrullus vulgaris	Watermelon
Punica granatum	Pomegranate
Ferona elephantum	Wood apple
Zizyphus jujuba	Jujube
Trichosanthes dioica	Pointed gourd
Cucurbita pepo	Field pumpkin
Juice prepared from these fruits can be consumed with rock salt and some spices.	
Vegetables:	
Scientific Name	English Name
China spinach	Amaranth
Amaranthus tristis	
Moringa oleifera	Drum stick
Trigonella foenum	Fenugreek
Peucedanum graveolens	Dill leaves
Hibiscus sabdariffa	Red sorrel
Spinacia olerecea	Spinach

Murraya koenigii	Curry leaves These leaves can be used while preparing curry
Mentha arvenis	Mint Chutney or sauce prepared from mint can be consumed with some spices.
Zizyphus jujuba	Leaves of zizyphus
Brassica oleracea	Cabbage
Non Leafy Vegetables:	
Embelica officinale	Indian gooseberry
Momordica charantia	Bitter gourd
Langeria vulgaris	Bottle gourd
Cyamopsis psoralioides	Cluster bean
Cala)ush Cucumber	Cucumber
Luffa aegyptiaca	
Abelmoschus esculentus	Ladies finger or okra
Luffa Koshataki	Ridge gourd
Trichosanthes anguina	Snake gourd
Solanum melongena	Brinjal gourd or egg plant only roasted brinjals should be consumed
Roots and Tubers:	
Beta vulgaris	Beet root
Daucus carota	Carrot
Amorpophallus paniculatus	Yam
Allium cepa	Onion Roasted onions helps to lose weight. It can be used to prepare chutney or sauce.
Raphanus sativus	Radish
Nuts and oil seeds:	
Carthamus tinctorius	Safflower seeds
Halianthus annus	Sunflower seeds
Oils collected from these seeds being light should be used to cook food.	
Cereal or Millets:	
Hordeum vulgare	Barley
Pennisetum typhoideum	Bajra
Andropogon sorghum	Jawar or Kalfir corn or Great millet
Zea mays	Maize or Corn
Elucine coracana	Ragi
These can be used to prepare chapati or bread. It is advocated to get millet roasted before its use.	
Pulses:	

Cicer arietinum	Bengal gram or Chick pea
Dolichos lablab	Flat bean or Goa bean
Phaseolus mungo	Green gram
Dolichos biflorus	Horse gram
Lens esculenta	Lentil Dal
Spices:	
Elettaria cadamomum	Cardamom
Ferula asafoetida	Asafoetida
Cumimum cymihym	Cumin seeds
Allium sativum	Garlic
Zingibar officinale	Ginger
Piper nigrum	Pepper
Curcuma longa	Turmeric
Brasica nigra	Black mustard seeds
Cinamomum zeylanicum	Cinamon
Capsicum aunum	Chillies
Miscellaneous:	
	Buttermilk (with watery consistency)
	Hot water should be consumed when one feels thirsty
	Chicken should be preferred over red meat
	Cow's milk
	Small sized fish can be consumed.
	Honey Honey with water taken in the morning helps to lose weight.

Donts

Scientific Name	English Name
Fruits:	
Musa sapientum	Banana
Anacardium occidentale	Cashew Fruit
Annona squamosa	Custard apple
Phonenix dactylifera	Dates
Ficus carica	Fig
Vitis venifera	Grapes
Artocarpus integrifolia	Jack fruit
Citrus Fruits:	
Mangifera indica	Mango
Farigaria vesca	Strawberry

Vegetables:	
Asparagus sarmentosus	
Asparagus officinalis	
Cucurbita maxima	Pumpkin
Glycine soja	Soyabean
Bennicapa hispida	Ash gourd or white gourd melon
Asparagus adsiendens	
Solanum nigrum	Garden-night-shade
Lepidum sativum	Watercress or Garden cress
Roots and Tubers:	
Solanum tuberosum	Potato
Ipomoea batatas	Sweet potato
Nuts:	
Prunus amygdalus	Almond
Anacardium occidentale	Cashew nut
Arachis hypogaea	Groundnut/ Peanut
Juglans regia	Walnut
Trapa bispinosa	Water chest nut
Oils:	
Arachic occidentale	Groundnut oil
	Sesame oil
	Butter
	Cheese
	Mayonnaise
Cereal:	
Triticum sativum	Wheat
Oryza sativa	Rice
Pulses:	
Phaseolus radiatus	Black gram
Miscellaneous:	
Sagus leavus	Sago

Prameha (Diabetes)

Diabetes is a common ailment in this modern era. Consumption of heavy, unctuous food and lack of exercise are the prime causative factor for diabetes. According to Ayurveda 'meda dhatu' is primarily affected in diabetes. It has classified diabetes into 20 types depending upon its manifestations. The main key for diabetes control is proper exercise and balanced diet. For better results, weight should be reduced in obese patients primarily. Polyuria (excessive urination) and polydipsia (excessive thirst) are the major symptoms observed.

Dos

English Name	Scientific Name
Fruits:	
Banana	*Musa sapientum*
Jambul fruit	*Eugenia jambulina*
Cluster fig	*Ficus glomerata*
Guava	*Psidium guyava*
Lime	*Citrus acida*
Pomegranate	*Punica granatum*
Wood apple	*Ferona elephantum*
Jujube	*Zizyphus jujuba*
Vegetables:	
Agathi	*Sesbenia grandiflora*
Amarnath	*Amaranthus tristis*
Amla or Indian gooseberry	*Emblica officinalis*
Bathua leaves white goose foot	*Chenopodium album*
Bengal gram leaves	*Cicer arietinum*
Mint	*Mentha sylvestris*
Coriander leaves	*Coriandrum sativum*
Fenugreek	*Trigonella foenum graeceum*
Hermaphrodite amaranth	*Amaranthus tenipolins*
Indian sorrel	*Oxalis corniculata*
Cabbage	*Brasica oleraseb capita*
Carrot leaves	*Daucus carota*
Cauliflower	*Brassica botrytis*
Cluster bean	*Cyamopsis psoralioides*
Celery leaves	*Apium graveolens*
Curry leaves	*Murraya koenigii*
Dill leaves	*Peucedanum graveolens*
Drumstick leaves	*Moringa oleifera*
Gotukola	*Centella asiatica*

Bitter gourd	*Momordica charantia*
Bottle gourd	*Langeria vulgaris*
French beans	*Phaseolus vulgaris*
Red sorrel	*Hibiscus sabdariffa*
Small caltrops	*Boerrhavia asiatica*
Snake gourd	*Trichosanthus anguina*
Spinach	*Spinacia olerecea*
Roots and Tubers:	
Beet root	*Beta vulgaris*
Carrot	*Daucus carota*
Onion	*Allium cepa*
Yam	*Dioscorea bulbifera*
Radish	*Raphanus sativus*
Nuts:	
Coconut	*Cocus nucifera*
Pistachio nut	*Pistacia vera*
Oils:	
Safflower oil	*Carthamus tinctorius*
Sunflower oil	*Helianthus annus*
Castor oil	*Ricinus communis*
Cereals or Millets:	
Bajra	*Pennisetum typhoidicum*
Barley	*Hordeum vulgare*
Jowar	*Sorghum vulgare*
Maize	*Zea mays*
Ragi	*Elucine coracana*
Pulses:	
Bengal gram	*Cicer arietinum*
Green gram	*Phaseolus mungo*
Horse gram	*Dolichos biflorus*
Flat bean or Goa bean	*Dolichos lablab*
Lentil	*Lens esculenta*
Red gram	*Cajanus indicus*
Spices:	
Asafoetida	*Ferula foetida*
Black mustard seeds	*Brasica nigra*
Cardamom	*Elettaria cardamomum*
Chillies	*Capsicum aunum*
Cinnamon	*Cinamomum zeylanicum*
Clove	*Eugenia caryophyllata*
Coriander seeds	*Coriandrum sativum*

Cumin seeds	*Cuminum cyminum*
Garlic	*Allium sativum*
Ginger	*Zingiber officinale*
Bishop's weeds	*Carum roxburghianum*
Pepper	*Piper nigrum*
Turmeric	*Curcuma longa*
Miscellaneous:	
Betel leaf	*Piper betel*
Cow's milk	
Butter milk	
Plain butter	
Honey	

Donts

English Name	Scientific Name
Fruits:	
Custard apple	*Annona squamosa*
Dates	*Phoenix dactylifera*
Mango	*Mangifera indica*
Jack fruit	*Artocarpus integrifolia*
Grape raisins	*Vitis vinifera*
Cherry	*Prunus cerasus*
Raspberry	*Rubus lasiocarpus*
Orange	*Citrus reticulata*
Palmyra palm	*Borasus flabelli formis*
Pineapple	*Ananas sativus*
Strawberry	*Farigaria vesca*
Pear	*Pyrus communis*
Tomato	*Lycopersicum esculentum*
Peach	*Prunus persica*
Vegetables:	
Spinach	*Spinacia olerecea*
Water cress or Garden cress	*Lepidum sativum*
Asaparagus	*Asaparagus racemosus*
Mustard leaves	*Brasica nigra*
Double beans	*Faba vulgaris*
Brinjal gourd	*Solanum melongena*
Broad beans	*Faba vulgaris*
Pumpkin	*Cucurbita maxima*
Ladies finger or Okra	*Hibiscus esculenthus*

Soybean	*Glycine soja*
Roots and Tubers:	
Sweet potato	*Ipomoea batatas*
Nuts:	
Cashew nut	*Anacardium occidentale*
Almond	*Prunus amygdalus*
Walnut	*Juglans regia*
Water chestnut	*Trapa bispinosa*
Oils:	
Ground nut oil	*Arachis hypogaea*
Cereals or Millets:	
Wheat	*Triticum sativum*
Pulses:	
Black gram	*Phaseolus radiatus*
Spices	
Tamarind	*Tamarindus indica*
Miscellaneous:	
Jaggery	
Curds Jaggery and curds are of the basic causative factors of diabetes.	
Sago	*Sagus leavus*
Sugar cane	*Sacchrum officinarum*
Yeast	*Cervisi actermeutum*
Cheese	
Alcohol In diabetes overall strength of the body is reduced. Alcohol consumption further vitiates the condition.	
Sweet. Sour and salty tastes in excess	
Red meat	

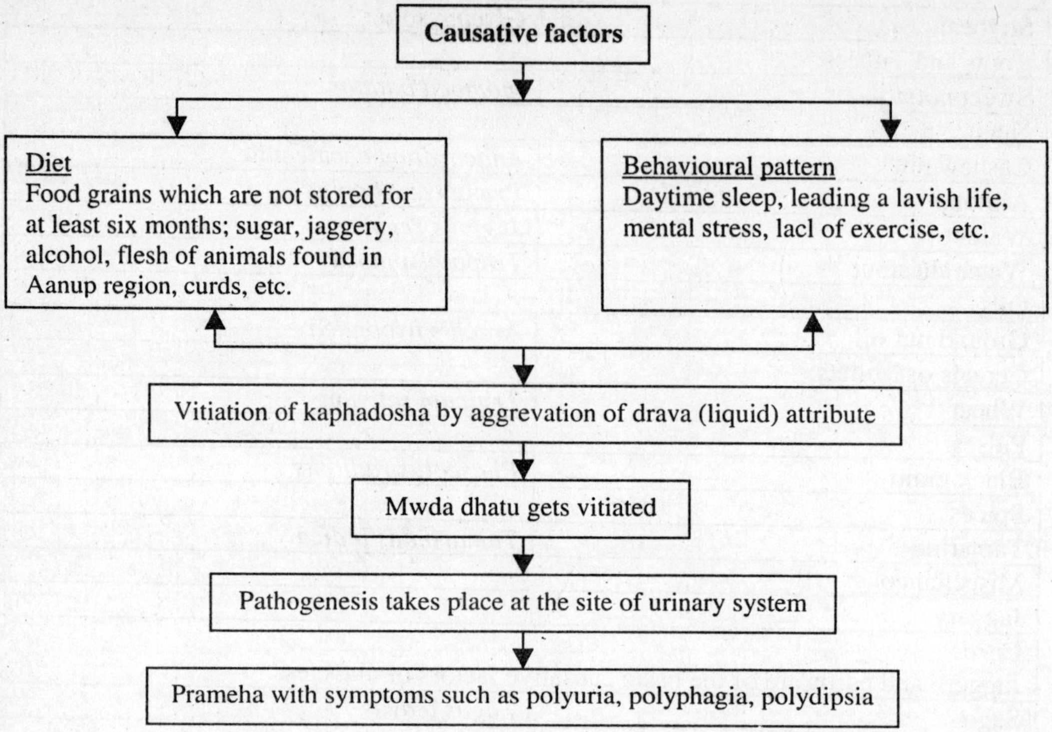
Causative factors
Diet
Food grains which are not stored for at least six months; sugar, jaggery, alcohol, flesh of animals found in Aanup region, curds, etc.
Behavioural pattern
Daytime sleep, leading a lavish life, mental stress, lacl of exercise, etc.
Vitiation of kaphadosha by aggrevation of drava (liquid) attribute
Mwda dhatu gets vitiated
Pathogenesis takes place at the site of urinary system
Prameha with symptoms such as polyuria, polyphagia, polydipsia

Urinary Calculus

This disorder of urinary system requires a proper diet pattern to help disintegrate the calculus. Following a regular diet pattern is also helpful in those who have undergone surgical removal of the calculus; to avoid the recurrence. Ayurveda suggests some fruits, vegetables and cuisine that helps to disintegrate the calculus as well as to flush it out in case of small sized calculus. This depends upon the size and the number of calculii.

Dos

English Name	Scientific Name
Fruits:	
Jack fruit	*Artocarpus integrifolia*
Coconut	*Coconut and its water*
Can be consumed according to the thirst. Paste of flowers of coconut in water with yavakshar (carbonate of potash) helps to disintegrate calculus.	
Watermelon	*Citrullus vulgaris*
Banana	*Musa sapientum*
Palmyra palm	*Borassus flabelli formis*
Grape raisins	*Witis vinifera*
Stargoose berry	*Cicco disticha*
This is a kind of amla, sour in taste. This has the property to disintegrate calcullii.	
Fig	*Ficus carica*
Sugarcane	*Saccharum officinarum*
Sugarcane increases the quantity of urine which helps to flush out the disintegrated calculus or small sized calculus.	
Wood apple	*Ferona elephantum*
According to modern science, the leaves of this plant help to reduce the tendency of calculus formation.	
Amla or Indian goosberry	*Emblica officinale*
Vegetables:	
Tinde This vegetable disintegrates calculus as well as being diuretic in nature flushes out the particles of calculus.	
Amaranth or China spinach	*Amaranthus spinosus*
Coleus Armmaticus	*Didymocarpus pedicellata.*
Carrot leaves	*Daucus carota*
Coleus Armmaticus	*Didymocarpus pedicellata*
Country boaroge or Thick leaved coleus	
Coriander leaves	*Coriandrum sativum*
Non Leafy Vegetables:	
Ash gourd	*Benincassa hispida*

An year old ash gourd should be consumed. A sweet dish called "petha" is prepared from it.	
Snake gourd	*Trichosanthus anguina*
Cucumber	*Cucumis sativus*
Root & tubers:	
Radish	*Raphanus sativus*
Beet root	*Beta vulgaris*
Onion	*Allium cepa*
Oils & Ghees:	
Oils should be used in less quantity in preparation of food.	
Groundnut oil	
Coconut oil	
Ghee prepared from cows milk.	
Ghee prepared from lamb has the property to reduce urinary calculus.	
Cereal:	
Barley Barley water helps as a diuretic.	*Hordeum vulgare*
Rice	*Oryza sativa*
Wheat	*Triticum sativum*
Pulses:	
Horse gram	*Dolichos biflorus*
Green gram	*Phaseolus mungo*
Black gram	*Phaseolus radiatus*
Spices:	
Cardamom	*Elettaria cardamomum*
Both the varieties of cardamom help in the disorders of urinary bladder.	
Cinnamon	*Cinamomum zeylanicicum*
Cinnamon acts on all the disorders of urinary system.	
Clove	*Eugenia caryophyllata*
Coriander seeds	*Coriandrum sativum*
Ginger	*Zinziber officinale*
Ginger has the property to disintegrate the calculus. Chutney/ sauce can be prepared from ginger. Ginger can be used while preparing tea.	
Cumin	*Cumimum cyminym*
Cumin seeds are diuretic in nature and help to reduce urinary disorders	
Seeds of carrot	*Daucus carota*
Seeds of carrot disintegrate the calculus and flush it out. Chutney/ sauce containing all the above spices can be prepared.	
Bishop's weeds	*Carum roxburghianum*
Miscellaneous:	
Eggs of birds habitant of desert have the	

property of disintegration of calculus.	
Cow's urine	
Indian short	*Canna edulis*

Donts

Dry, heavy food, wrong combinated food should be strictly avoided.

English Name	Scientific Name
Fruits:	
Jambul fruit	*Eugenia jambolana*
Wood apple	*Ferona elephantum*
Bokhera plum	*Cherry plum*
Pineapple	*Ananas sativus*
Peach	*Prunus persica*
Tomato	*Lycopersicum esculentum*
Vegetables:	
Fenugreek	*Trigonella foenum graeceum*
Red sorrel	*Hibiscus sabdariffa*
Keshari leaves	*Lathyrus sativa*
Non leafy vegetables:	
Brinjal gourd	*Solanum melongena*
Bitter gourd	*Mormordica charantia*
Calabush cucumber	*Luffa aegyptiaca*
Pumpkin	*Cucurbita maxima*
Ridge gourd	*Luffa acutengula*
Root and Tubers:	
Great leaved caledium	*Erum indicum*
Potato	*Solanum tuberosum*
Yarn	*Dioscorea bulbifera*
Oils:	
Mustard oil	*Brasica nigra*
Safflower oil	*Carthamus tinctorius*
Cereals and Millets:	
Chickling vetch	*Lathiyrus sativus*
Pulses:	
Bengal gram	*Cicer arietinum*
Field pea	*Pisum sativum*
Spices:	
Asafoetida	*Ferula foetida*
Black mustard seeds	*Brasica nigra*

Chillies	*Capsicum aunum*
Consumption of all the other spices in excess is proscripted.	
Miscellaneous:	
Areca nut	Areca catechu
Vinegar	

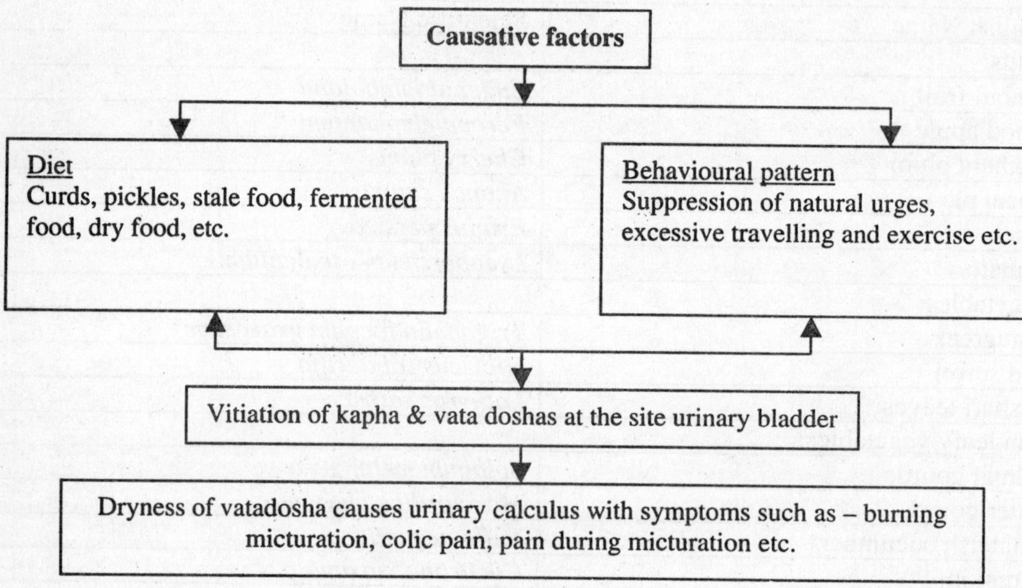

<u>Vatavyadhi</u> (various aches in the body)

The ache or pain caused in any part of the body is one of the signs of vitiation of vata dosha. Vata dosha when vitiated may give rise to various disorders such as spondylosis, spondylitis, joint pain, palsies, prolapse of vertebral disc etc. Ayurveda studies all these disorders under one name 'VATAVYADHI' and aims at alleviation of vata dosha. Some eating habits and food items have inclination towards elevation of vata dosha, while some help to alleviate the vata dosha and relieve pain.

Consumption of proper amount of unctuous material and warm food certainly helps to reduce the level of vata dosha. Here are some food items which are beneficial in vatavyadhi.

Dos

English Name	Scientific Name
Fruits:	
Apple	*Pyrus malus*
Apricot	*Prunus armeniaca*
Banana	*Musa sapientum*
Mango	*Mangifera indica*
Cashew fruit	*Anacardium occidentale*
Custard apple	*Annona squamosa*
Dates	*Phoenix dactylifera*
Cluster fig	*Ficus glomerata*
Grapes Grapes are beneficial in especially gout.	*Vitis vinifera*
Guava	*Psidium guyava*
Jack fruit	*Artocarpus integrifolia*
Lime	*Citrus acida*
Orange	*Citrus reticulata*
Sweet orange	*Citrus aurantium*
Citron	*Citrus medica*
Pomegranate	*Punica granatum*
Vegetables:	
Bathua leaves	*Chenopodium album*
Celery leaves	*Apium graveolens*
Coriander leaves	*Coriandrum sativum*
Curry leaves	*Murraya koenigii*
Drumstick leaves	*Moringa oleifera*
Garden cress leaves or water cress leaves	*Lepidum sativum*
Ladies finger or okra	*Hibiscus esculenthus*

Mint	*Mentha arvenis*
Asparagus	*Asparagus officinalis*
Indian gooseberry	*Emblica officinalis*
Ash gourd	*Benincasa hispida*
Cucumber	*Cucumis sativus*
Calabush cucumber	*Luffa aegyptiaca*
Snake gourd	*Tricosanthes anguina*
Roots and Tubers:	
Beet root	*Beta vulgaris*
Carrot	*Daucus carota*
Nuts:	
Almonds	*Prunus amygdalus*
Cashew nut	*Anacardium occidentale*
Coconut	*Cocus nucifera*
Walnut	*Juglans regia*
Oils:	
Sesame oil	*Sesamum indicum*
Groundnut oil	*Archic hypogaca*
Cereals or Millets:	
Rice grains	*Oryza sativa*
Wheat	*Triticum sativum*
Wheat gives strength to the bone tissue and relieves vata.	
Pulses:	
Black gram	*Phaseolus radiatus*
Green gram	*Phaseolus mungo*
Preparation of pulses should be consumed with ghee or oils as they are ununctuous.	
Spices:	
Asafoetida	*Ferula asafoetida*
Cardamom	*Elettaria cardamomum*
Coriander seeds	*Coriandrum sativum*
Cumin seeds	*Cumimum cyminym*
Garlic	*Allium sativum*
Ginger	*Zingiber officinale*
Bishop's weeds	*Carum roxburghianum*
Tamarind	*Tamarindus indica*
Turmeric	*Curcuma longa*
Mustard seeds	*Brasica nigra*
Dry ginger	*Zinziber officinale*
All the spices are good pain relievers.	
Miscellaneous:	

Cow's ghee	
Unsalted butter	
Cow's milk	
Sheep's milk and ghee	
Fish	

Donts

English Name	Scientific Name
Fruits:	
Jambul fruit	*Eugenia jambolana*
Palmyra palm	*Borassus flabelli formis*
Water melon	*Citrullus vulgaris*
Bokhera plum	*Cherry plum*
Lakuch	*Artocarpus lacoochaii*
Mango	*Mangifera indica*
Unripe green mangoes elevate vata dosha.	
Stargoose berry	*Cicco disticha*
Water caltrop	*Trapa bispinosa*
Narrow leaved sepistun	*Cordia myza*
Fig	*Ficus carica*
Vegetables:	
Agathi	*Aeschynomene grandiflora*
Marish	*Amaranthus tricalar*
Pattashak	*Ipomoea reprama*
Kessoor	*Scripus kessoor*
Hermaphrodite amarnath	*Amaranthus oleraceus*
Acute angled cucumber or ridge gourd	*Luffa acutengula*
Pubesceunt cucumber	*Cucumis babeseens*
Brinjal	*Solanum melongena*
Spinach	*Spinasia oleracea*
Bitter gourd	*Mormodica charantia*
Capsicum	
French beans	*Phaseolus vulgaris*
Roots and Tubers:	
Potato	*Solanum tuberosum*
Sweet potato	*Ipomoea batatas*
Yam	*Dioscorea bulbifera*
Nuts:	
Betel nut	*Areca catechu*
Oils:	

Safflower oil	*Carthamus tinctorius*
Sunflower oil	*Halianthus annus*
<u>Cereals and Millets</u>:	
Barley	*Hordeum vulgare*
Jowar	*Sorghum vulgare*
Millet	*Panicum miliari*
Shyamak	*Panicum frumentaceum*
Punctured paspalum	*Paspalum serobiculatum*
<u>Pulses</u>:	
Bengal gram	*Cicer arietinum*
Flat bean or Goa bean	*Dolicohs lablab*
Lentil	*Lens esculenta*
Red gram	*Cajanus indicus*
Aconite leaved kidney beans	*Phaseolus aconitum*
Field pea	*Pisum sativum*
Chickling vetch	*Lathiyrus sativus*
This should never be consumed as it has great potential to vitiate vata dosha. Regular intake of it may create anatomical deformity.	
<u>Miscellaneous</u>:	
Alcohol Alcohol consumption relives pain temporarily but its regular intake certainly vitiates vata and pitta.	

<u>Discussion</u>:

In this modern era, people are very conscious about their weight and physique. Many times to reduce or maintain the weight, intake of unctuousness is strictly restricted which, leads to vitiation of vata dosha. This vitiation may generate various disorders like spondylosis, osteoarthritis, muscular pain etc.

Our body needs certain amount of unctuousness for the smooth functioning. Ayurveda strongly recommends intake of cow's ghee in regular diet as it supplies proper amount of unctuousness to the body. It can be consumed in almost all the diseases by following regular rules of diet.

According to the modern dietetics cow's ghee has omega 3 or N-3 cells which increases the HDL and it is known that HDL is good for the cardiac muscles. Cow's ghee does not increase the cholesterol level, and can be consumed following regular routes of diet.

Miscellaneous in Disease and Ahar

1. Dietary Regimen after Surgery

Internal medication and local applications are usually prescribed after minor and major surgeries. Ayurveda recommends a specific dietary regimen for post operative care, as improper diet may disturb the process of wound healing.

Barley, wheat, a variety of rice which is harvested after 60 days (shashtik), lentils, green gram, tuvarak (Hydnocarpus laurifolia), radish (tender), brinjal, hermaphrodite amaranth (Amaranthus oleraceus), white goose foot or bathua leaves (Chenopodium album), bitter gourd, serpent gourd (Trichosanthus dioica), rock salt, pomegranate, Indian gooseberry (Emblica officinalis), cow's ghee, lukewarm water, flesh of animals of jangal desha, etc. can be consumed.

Newly harvested grains, sesame seeds, black gram, alcohol, preparations of milk, preparations of sugarcane, cold, sour, salty, and pungent food stuffs etc. should not be consumed.

2. Pregnancy

Pregnancy is a very delicate condition in a woman's life that needs proper nourishment for the health of the mother and the baby. Physical and mental wellbeing of the mother results in a healthy child.

During pregnancy the mother has to supply required nutrients to the foetus and her body as well. In this period body traverses through various anatomical as well as physiological changes which may give symptoms like - nausea, vomiting, loss of appetite etc. With some changes in daily diet and behaviour pattern, one can easily overcome these symptoms and make pregnancy the most pleasuresome phase of the life. Ayurveda recommends light but nutritious diet with the dominance of 'satva' attribute in it. Such a diet gets easily digested and nourishes the body as well as mind.

Dos

English Name	Scientific Name
Fruits:	
Apple	*Pyrus malus*
Banana Banana should be consumed with honey or home made ghee.	*Musa sapientum*
Cherry	*Prunus cerasus*
Custard apple	*Annona squamosa*
Dates	*Phoenix dactylifera*
Fig	*Ficus carica*
Cluster fig	*Ficus glomerata*
Grapes	*Vitis vinifera*
Guava	*Psidium guyava*
Jackfruit Ripen jackfruit should be consumed.	*Artocarpus integrifolia*
Pomegranate	*Punica granatum*
Sweet orange	*Citrus aurantium*
Sugar cane	*Saccharum officinarum*
Mango	*Mangifera indica*
Melon	*Cucumis melo*
Peach	*Prunus persica*
Strawberry	*Farigaria vesca*
Lime	*Citrus acida*
Amla or Indian gooseberry	*Emblica officinalis*
Vegetables:	
Ash gourd or white pumpkin	*Benincasa hispida*

Bottle gourd	*Langeria vulgaris*
Calabash cucumber	*Luffa aegyptiaca*
Cauliflower	*Bassica botrytis*
Cluster bean	*Cyamopsis psoralioides*
Cucumber	*Cucumis sativus*
Okra or Ladies finger	*Abelmoschus esculentus*
Green peas	*Pisum sativum*
Pumpkin	*Cucurbita maxima·*
Snake gourd	*Trichosanthes anguina*
Soyabean	*Glycine soja*
White goose foot or Bathua leaves	*Chenopodium album*
Red malabar night shods	*Bassela rubra* or *Bassela alba*
Cabbage	*Brasica oleraseb capita*
Carrot leaves	*Daucus carota*
Celery leaves	*Apium graveolens*
Coriander leaves	*Coriandrum sativum*
Curry leaves	*Murraya koenigii*
Garden cress or water cress	*Lepidum sativum*
Asparagus	*Asparagus officinalis*
Small caltrops	*Boerrhavia diffusa*
Gotukola	*Centella asiatica*
Roots and Tubers:	
Beet	*Beta vulgaris*
Carrot	*Daucus carota*
Beet and carrot should be regularly consumed. Whereas seeds of carrot are strongly contraindicated in pregnancy.	
Onion	*Allium cepa*
Potato	*Solanum tuberosum*
Sweet potato	*Ipomoea batatas*
Yam	*Dioscorea bulbifera*
Nuts:	
Almond	*Prunus amygdalus*
Cashew nut	*Anacardium occidentale*
Coconut	*Cocus nucifera*
Walnut	*Juglans regia*
Pistachio nut	*Pistacia vera*
Groundnut	*Hypogaca arachic*
Oils:	
Sunflower oil	*Helianthus annus*
Coconut oil	*Cocus nucifera*
Groundnut oil	*Hypogaca arachic*

Cereals or Millets:	
Rice	*Oryza sativa*
Maize	*Zea mays*
Ragi	*Elucine coracana*
Wheat	*Triticum sativum*
Pulses:	
Bengal gram	*Cicer arietinum*
Green gram	*Phaseolus mungo*
Lentil	*Lens esculenta*
Black gram	*Phaseolus radiatus*
Flat bean or Goa bean	*Dolichos lablab*
Red gram	*Cajanus indicus*
All the pulses may create flatulance and hence should be consumed with spices like ginger, garlic etc. and in less quantity.	
Spices:	
Asafoetida	*Ferula foetida*
Cinnamon	*Cinamomum zeylanicum*
Coriander seeds	*Coriandrum sativum*
Garlic	*Allium sativum*
Ginger	*Zinziber officinale*
Saffron	*Croci stigmata*
Bishop's weeds	*Carum roxburghianum*
Fennel seeds	*Foeniculum vulgare*
Black mustard seeds	*Brasica nigra*
Turmeric	*Curcuma longa*
Tamarind	*Tamarindus indica*
Miscellaneous:	
Cow's milk	
Plain butter	
Ghee (clarified butter)	
Butter milk	
Sago	*Sagus leavus*

Donts

English Name	Scientific Name
Fruits:	
Papaya	*Carica papaya*
Papaya is strongly contraindicated in pregnancy	
Pineapple	*Ananas sativus*
Citron	*Citrus medica*

Wood apple	*Ferona elephantum*
Vegetables:	
Agathi	*Aeschynomene grandiflora*
Bengal gram leaves	*Cicer arientinum*
Drum stick leaves	*Moringa oleifera*
Dill leaves	*Peucedanum graveolens*
French beans	*Phaseolus vulgaris*
Brinjal	*Solanum melongena*
Broad beans	*Faba vulgaris*
Ridge gourd	*Luffa acutengula*
Roots and Tubers:	
Radish	*Raphanus sativus*
Nuts:	
Nutmeg	*Myristica fragrans*
Oils:	
Castor oil	*Ricinus communis*
Mustard oil	*Brasica nigra*
Cereals and Millets:	
Barley	*Hordeum vulgare*
Pulses:	
Horse gram	*Dolichos biflorus*
Spices:	
Chillies	*Capsicum aunum*
Clove	*Eugenia caryophyllata*
Pepper	*Piper nigrum*
Cardamom	*Elettaria cardamomum*
Cumin seeds	*Cuminum cyminum*
Miscellaneous:	
Areca nut/ Betel nut	*Areca catechu*
Betel leaves	*Piper betel*
Lime stone	*Calcium hydroxide*
Vinegar	
Yeast	*Cervisi actermeutum*
Ajinomoto	
Colustrum of animals	
Red meat	
Excess of salt should be avoided	
Wine and alcohols are strongly contraindicated.	

3. **Post natal care/ Perpeureum**

This is the period after delivery of the baby which needs proper attention and care. Delivery of a baby is a stressful activity for the mother and the baby as well. It causes immense vataprakopa which needs to be alleviated by a specific diet. This diet also promotes the process of lactation.

Negligence towards the health may result in fatigue, fever, joint pain, obesity, loss of appetite etc. To alleviate the vata dosha, healthy, nutritious, unctuous but light diet, fomentation, proper diets are supplementary to restore the health. In the early stage of life, breast milk is the only source of food for the baby and good amount of milk certainly provides the baby the healthy nourishment.

Dos

English Name	Scientific Name
Fruits:	
Asiatic greevia	*Greevia asiatica*
Apple	*Pyrus malus*
Banana	*Musa sapientum*
Cherries	*Prunus cerasus*
Coconut Coconut water can be taken.	*Cocus nucifera*
Dates	*Phoenix dactylifera*
Jack fruit	*Artocarpus integrifolia*
Jambul fruit	*Eugenia jambulina*
Cluster fig	*Ficus glomerata*
Elloopa tree	*Bassia longifolia*
Fig	*Ficus carica*
Grapes Only sweet grapes should be consumed.	*Vitis vinifera*
Lime	*Citrus acida*
Mustard tree of scripture	*Salvadora parsica*
Obtuse leaved mimusops	*Mimusops hexendra*
Orange	*Citrus reticulata*
Papaya	*Carica papaya*
Pomegranate	*Punica granatum*
Peach	*Prunus persica*
Pear	*Pyrus communis*
Raspberry	*Rubus lasiocarpus*
Strawberry	*Farigaria vesca*
Wood apple	*Ferona elephantum*

Jujube	*Zizyphus jujuba*
Vegetables:	
Asparagus	*Asparagus officinalis*
Ash gourd or White gourd	*Benincasa hispida*
Indian gooseberry	*Emblica officinalis*
Bathua leaves	*Chenopodium album*
Bengal gram leaves	*Cicer arietinum*
Garden cress or Water cress leaves	*Lepidum sativum*
Mint	*Mentha sylvestris*
Coriander leaves	*Coriandrum sativum*
Fenugreek	*Trigonella foenum graeceum*
Hermaphrodite amaranth	*Amaranthus tenipolins*
Cabbage	*Brasica oleraseb capita*
Carrot leaves	*Daucus carota*
Cauliflower	*Bassica botrytis*
Celery leaves	*Apium graveolens*
Curry leaves	*Murraya koenigii*
Drumstick leaves	*Moringa olefera*
Small caltrops	*Boerrhavia asiatica*
Spinach	*Spinacia olerecea*
Oils:	
Groundnut oil	
Sunflower oil	*Helianthus annus*
Castor oil	*Ricinus communis*
Cereals or Millets:	
Bajra	*Pennisetum typhoidicum*
Barley	*Hordeum vulgare*
Jowar	*Sorghum vulgare*
Maize	*Zea mays*
Rice	*Oryza sativa*
Ragi	*Elucine coracana*
Pulses:	
Green gram	*Phaseolus mungo*
Spices:	
Asafoetida	*Ferula foetida*
Black mustard seeds	*Brasica nigra*
Cardamom	*Elettaria cardamomum*
Cinnamon	*Cinamomum zeylanicum*
Clove	*Eugenia caryophyllata*
Coriander seeds	*Coriandrum sativum*
Cumin seeds	*Cuminum cyminum*

Fennel seeds	*Foeniculum vulgare*
Folia malabathy	*Cinnamomum tamala*
Garlic	*Allium sativum*
Ginger	*Zingiber officinale*
Bishop's weeds	*Carum roxburghianum*
Nutmeg	*Myristica fragrans*
Pepper	*Piper nigrum*
Turmeric	*Curcuma longa*
Miscellaneous:	
Cow's ghee Consumption of ghee is very essential to alleviate vata and accelerate the process of lactation.	
Cow's milk	
Butter milk	
Plain butter	
Edible gum	
Honey	
Water cress or Garden cress seeds Porridge prepared with watercress seeds is very beneficial for lactation.	*Lepidum sativum*

Donts

English Name	Scientific Name
Fruits:	
Sugarcane	*Saccharum officinarum*
Stargooseberry	*Phyllanthus distincha*
Mango	*Mangifera indica*
Jack fruit	*Artocarpus integrifolia*
Jasmine flowered carrissa	*Carrissa cordandal*
Water caltrop	*Trapa bispinosa*
Mulberry	*Morus indica*
Poison nut	*Strychnus nux vomica*
Palmyra palm	*Borasus flabelli formis*
Lakooch	*Artocarpus lacoochaii*
Custard apple	*Annona squamosa*
Mango, jack fruit and custard apple increases the production of milk but these fruits being heavy to digest should not be consumed in the first month of post natum.	
Vegetables:	
Red sorrel	*Hibiscus sabdariffa*
Mustard leaves	*Brasica nigra*

Bitter gourd	*Momordica charantia*
Calabush cucumber	*Luffa aegyptiaca*
Cluster bean	*Cyamopsis psoralioides*
Cucumber	*Cucumis sativus*
Double beans	*Faba vulgaris*
Brinjal gourd	*Solanum melongena*
Peas	*Pisum sativum*
Broad beans	*Faba vulgaris*
Pumpkin	*Cucurbita maxima*
Ridge gourd	*Luffa acutangula*
Ladies finger or Okra	*Hibiscus esculenthus*
Snake gourd	*Trichosanthes anguina*
Soyabean	*Glycine soja*
Roots and Tubers:	
Beet root	*Beta vulgaris*
Carrot	*Daucus carota*
Colocasia	*Colocasia antiquorum*
Onion	*Allium cepa*
Potato	*Solanum tuberosum*
Radish	*Raphanus sativus*
Sweet potato	*Ipomoea batatas*
Yam	*Dioscorea bulbifera*
Nuts:	
Cashew nut	*Anacardium occidentale*
Almond	*Prunus amygdalus*
Ground nut	*Arachis hypogaea*
Pistachionut	*Pistacia vera*
Walnut	*Juglans regia*
Water chestnut	*Trapa bispinosa*
Oils:	
Sesame oil	*Sesamum indicum*
Olive oil	*Olea europea*
Safflower oil	*Carthamus tinctorius*
Cereals or Millets:	
Wheat	*Triticum sativum*
Pulses:	
Bengal gram	*Cicer arietinum*
Black gram	*Phaseolus radiatus*
Green gram	*Phaseolus mungo*
Horse gram	*Dolichos biflorus*
Flat bean or Goa bean	*Dolichos lablab*

Lentil dal	*Lens esculenta*
Red gram	*Cajanus indicus*
<u>Spices</u>:	
Chillies	*Capsicum aunum*
<u>Miscellaneous</u>:	
Areca nut	
Curds	
Sago	*Sagus leavus*
Betel leaves	*Piper betel*
Yeast	*Cervisi actermeutum*
Vinegar	
Hard cheese	
Buffalo's milk	
Fish	
Meat	
Salted butter	
Fermented food stuffs	

4. **Sansarjan Kram**

Panchakarma is a specialised branch of Ayurvedic medicine in which vitiated doshas are eliminated out of the body by various procedures.

Vaman, virechan, basti, nasya and raktamokshan are the five procedures included in Panchakarma Therapy. During and after these procedures the levels of doshas are changed; which lead to decrease in the power of agni. This power has to be increased gradually by supplying the food which is easy to digest and also beneficial in alleviation of remaining doshas. This particular dietetic regimen is called as 'Sansarjan Kram'.

Diet after Panchakarma: The post Panchakarma dietary regimen is called as sansarjan kram. During vaman and virechana karma there is much stress on Annavaha srotas and the digestive fire gets slowed. Hence it is advised to follow the dietetic regimen with peya, vilepi etc. in three, two or one mealtime respectively according to the degree of evacuation like superior, medium or inferior.

As little finger kindled gradually with grass, cow dung etc. becomes great, stable and all digesting the internal fire of the evacuated one does like with peya etc. says charaka. Some peculiarities of sansarjan krama:

1. The duration of sansarjan krama depends on the degree of samshodhana (the time elimination of doshas).
2. The quantity of the preparation depends on the appetite of patient.
3. Sansarjan kram should begin with liquid gruel (Mandayukta Yavagu and end with Odana with meat soup irrespective of duration of sansarjan krama.
4. A specific sequence of Rasa should be followed while preparing the gruels etc.

Though the sansarjan krama depends on the degree of samshodhana, charakacharya described the full regimen useful in superior degree of evacuation.

Mandayukta yavagu i.e. scummy gruel of red rice is advised for first three meals. A paste like preparation of red rice with or without unctuous substance and salt is advised for next three meals. Cooked red rice with green gram soup and little unctuous substance and salt is advised for next three meals and cooked red rice with birds meat soup and salt is advised for last three meals.

Sushrut has advised to consume 1/4th quantity of the daily requirement of a person; e.g. if a person consumes 400 gm of rice for a meal. Then 100 gm of rice is recommended for these preparations.

The Importance of Sequence:

In Manda the proportion of rice and water is 1:14, in yavagu it is 1:6, oin vilepi, it is 1:4 and in odana it should be 1:5.

For first three meal 'Mandayukta Yavagu" i.e. a scummy liquid gruel of red rice is advised. Looking at the proportion of water and rice this preparation must be a liquid preparation. This preparation includes liquid food containing solids which are not very difficult to digest.

In 4th, 5th and 6th meal vilepi i.e. a paste like preparation is advised. In this preparation particle size of the rice becomes very small.

In 7th, 8th and 9th meal odana along with dilute green gram soup, liitle unctuous substance and salt is advised. This becomes nutritionally adequate because of the addition of green gram soup. This preparation is also soft in texture and consistancy, easy to chew and contains low roughage.

In 10th, 11th, and 12th meal odana alongwith birds meat soup with little salt is advised. Birds meat soup is a good source of nourishment and after this, patient can switch over to his routine diet.

SLOKAS

Peace of mind improves appetite and helps in digestion. There are various shlokas to be enchanted before having food. Just listening to these shlokas during meals also help you to achieve the peace of mind.

There are a nunmber of shlokas on this subject in various ancient Indian literatures. Some of them are compiled here. These describe the customs and traditions of Indian dietary habits and also various environmental conditions suitable for consumption of food. Here *Sudra* does not stand for any caste or class of people but the unclean and darty people.

1.

स्त्रात्वा पूक्षाल्य पादौ च सूग्गन्धालंकृतः शुचिः ।

पञ्चयज्ञावशिष्टं तु भुङ्क्ते यः सोऽमृताशनः ॥

उपलिप्ते शुचौ देशे पादौ पूक्षाल्य वाग्यतः ।

प्राङ्मुखोऽन्नानि भुञ्जित शुचिः पठिमधिष्ठितः ॥

Snatva praksalya padau ca sraggandhalankrtah sucih /
pancayajnavasistan tu bhunkte yah so'mrtasanah //
Upalipte sucau dese padau praksalya vagyatah /
Prarimukhonnani sucih pithamadhisthitah //

Having taken a bath (after traversing muddy ground etc.) one should be pure by washing both feet, be adorned with flower garlands and sandal paste and then eat whatever remains after offering food in the five sacrifice like rites

I) offering in smarta fire
II) offering food to forefathers
III) vedic studies (naivedya)
IV) feeding guests and
V) scattering food (to beings like dogs, crows etc.); one eating such food eats ambrosia.

One should wash feet (outside the dining hall), be pure, sit on a flat stool (placed in) cowdung-smeared and (hence) pure place, be restrained in speech (silent) and face the east to take food.

2.

विशेद्भोजनभुमि तु सुपूक्षालितपाणिमान् ।

आसनस्थस्तु यो दर्पात् पडिक्तमध्ये उपस्पृशेत् ॥

स सर्वेषां तु यत्पापं तत् गृण्हाति नराधमः ।

तस्माद्बहिरूपस्पृश्य आचान्तः पूविशेत् गृहम् ॥

Vised bhojanabhumin tu supraksalitapaniman /
asanasthas tu yo darpat panktimadhye upasprset //
sa sarvesan tu yat papan tad grhnati naradhamah /
tasmad bahir upasprsya acantah pravised grham //

One should enter the dining hall, washing hands clean beforehand. He who after taking seat, through pride sips water right within the (dining) row, that wretched man receives the sin of all (eaters).

3.

उपलिप्य समे स्थाने शुचौ श्लक्ष्णासनान्विते ।

चतुरस्रं त्रिकोणं तु वर्त्तुलं चार्ध्दचन्द्रकम् ॥

कर्त्तव्यामानुपूर्वेण ब्रूाहमणादिषु मण्डलम् ॥

Upalipya same sthane#sucau slaksnasananvite /
caturasran trikonan tu vartulan cardhacandrakam //
kartavyamanupurvyena brahmanadisu mandalam //

A levelled pure ground should be smeared (with cowdung), then soft seats should be arranged. For Brahman etc. serially figures of rectangle, triangle, circle and semicircle should be drawn (in *rangavali*).

4.

बूहमरुद्रेन्द्रचन्द्रार्कवसवो मण्डलान्तरात् ।

निवेदितं नरैरन्नं तस्मात् गृण्हान्ति नान्यथा ॥

अकृत्वा मण्डलं ये तु भञ्जते ऽधमयोनयः ।

तेषां तु यक्षरक्षांसि हरन्त्यन्नस्य तदबलम् ॥

Brchma-rudrendra-candrarka-vasavo mandalantarat /
nivedin narair annan tasmad grhnanti nanyatha //

akrtva mandalam ye#tu bhunjate' dhamayonayah /
tesantu yaksaraksamsi harnty annasya tad balam //

Brahman, Rudra, Indra, Moon, Sun and eight Vasus partake food offered by men inside (geometrical) figures, not otherwise of lowly-born people who dine without drawing (geometrical) figures, the sap of food is snatched by (evil beings) Yaksa and Demons.

5.

नैकवस्त्रधरो नार्द्रपाणिपादो नरेश्वर ।

विशुद्धवदनः प्रीतो भुञ्जीत न विदिङ्मुख ॥

प्राङ्मुखोदङ्मुखो वापि नचैवान्यमना नरः ।
विदिङ्मुखः आग्नेयादिकोणाभिमुखः ॥

आयुष्यं प्राङ्मुखो भुङ्क्ते यशस्यं दक्षिणामुखः ।

श्रियं प्रत्यङ्मुखो भुङ्क्ते ऋतं भुङ्क्ते शुदङ्मुखः ॥

Naikavestredharo nardrapanipado naresvara /
visuddhavadanah prito bhunjita na vidinmukhah //
pranimukhodanmukho vapi, na caivanyamana narah /
ayusyam pranmukho bhunkte, yasasyan daksinamukhah /
sriyam pratyanmukho bhurikte, rtam bhunkte hyudanmukhah //

Oh king! One should not dine with one garment (i.e., dhoti) only, one should not eat without washing hands and feet, one should not dine facing intemediate directions (i.e., one should eat food with dhoti and uttariya, after washing hands and feet. One should not face the intermediate direction – intermediate means south-east etc (line 4))

One who dines facing the East, enjoys life.
One who dines facing the South, enjoys fame.
One who dines facing the West, enjoys wealth.
One who dines facing the North, enjoys truth.

6.

आर्द्रपादस्तु भुञ्जीयात् प्राङ्मुखश्चासने शुचौ ।

पादाभ्यां धरणी स्पृष्टवा पादेनैकेन वा पुनः ॥

Ardapadas tu bhunjiyat pranmukhas casane sucau /
padabhyan dharanim sprstva padenaikena va#punah //

One should moisten his feet, take a seat on a seat placed on (cow-dung) pure (ground), face the East and dine. He may touch the ground with both feet or one foot (while eating).

7.

सायम्प्रार्मनुष्याणामशनं देवनिर्मितम् ।

नान्तरा भोजनं कुर्यादग्निहोत्रसमो विधिः ॥

Sayam-pratar manusyanam asanan devanirmitam /
nantara bhojanan kuryad agnihotrasamo vidhih //

God has enjoined dining in the evening and morning. Taking food is as sacred as daily sacrifice (performed twice – evening and morning). Hence one should not eat food (extra) within these two times. Fruits are allowed (one should dine only twice a day).

8.

मनिभिर्द्विरशनमुक्तं विप्राणामन्त्यवासिनां नित्यम् ।

अहनि च तथा तमस्विन्यां सार्धप्रहरयामान्तः ॥

Munibhir dvir asanam uktam vipranam antyavasinan nityam /
ahani ca tatha tamasvinyam sardhapraharayamantah //

Sagas have always enjoined for Brahmins to untouchables (i.e. for all) dining twice (a day). One during day time and after 1 ½ *prahara* i.e. about 5 hours and 15 minutes.

9.

उपघातादृते दोषं नान्नस्योदीरयेत् बुधः ।

वीरमित्रोदयसयाहिणक शे ॥

Upaghatad rte dosa nannasyodirayed budhah //

A wise person should not find fault with food except offences (like touching of food by dogs, crows etc; sight of a women in menses, etc.).

10.

भूमौ पात्रं प्रतिष्ठाप्य यो भुङ्क्ते वाग्यतः शुचिः ।

भोजने भोजने नित्यं त्रिरात्रकलमश्नुते ॥

Bhumau patram pratisthapya yo bhunkte vagyatah sucih /
bhojane bhojane nityan triratraphalam asnute //

Pure (by bathing) restrained in speech (silently) one eats keeping the plate on ground. Such a person gets the reward for three day penance at each dining.

11.

न्यस्तपात्रस्तु भुञ्जीत पञ्चग्रासान् महामुने ।

शेषमुद्धृत्य भोक्तव्यं शूयतामत्र कारणम् ॥

Nyastapatras tu bhunjita pancagrasan mahamune /
sesam uddhrtya bhoktavyam sruyatam atra karanam //

Oh great sage, one should partake five morsels keeping the plate on ground. The rest of the food should be partaken after raising the plate. Hear the cause for this.

12.

विप्रुषां दोषसंस्पर्शः पादचैलरजस्तथा ।

सुखेन भुङ्क्ते विप्रोऽपि पितृर्थ तु न लुप्यते ॥

Viprusan dosasamsparsah padacailarajas tatha /
sukhena bhunkte vipro'pi pitrarthan tu na lupyate //

The unhygenic touch of saliva (from mouth), dust sticking to feet or both garments. Hence even a Brahmin should eat comfortably (raising the plate after five morsels). However placing on ground the plate of food for forefathers is not prohibited.

13.

प्राणेभ्यस्त्वथ पञ्चभ्यः स्वाहाप्रणवसंयुताः ।

पञ्चाहुतीस्तु जुहुयात् प्रलयाग्निनिभेषु च ॥

Pranebhyas tvatha pancabhyah svahapranavasamyutah /
pancahutis tu juhuyat pralayagninibhesu ca //

To the five pranas (prana, apana, vyana, udana samana), five oblations (one per each) with OM in the beginning and svaha in the end (OM samanaya svaha) should be offered because they are like fires at the time of dissolution of world.

14.

भोजनात्किंचिदन्नाद्यं धर्मराजाय वै बलिम् ।

दत्वाऽथ चित्रगुप्ताय प्रेतेभ्यश्चेदमुच्चरन् ॥

यत्र कचन संस्थानां क्षुत्तृषोपहतात्मनाम् ।

प्रेतानां तृप्तयेऽक्षय्यमिदमस्तु यथासुखम् ॥

Bhojanat kincid annadyan dharmarajaya vai balim /
dattvatha citraguptaya pretebhyas cedam uccaran //
yatra-kvaccna-samsthanan ksuttrsopahatatmanam /
pretanan trptaye ksayyamidam astu yathasukham //

From the food some portion to Yama (god of death) and Citragupta (accountant of Yama) should be offered. Pronouncing to all the departed, residing here and there, afflicted by hunger and thirst, let this (scattered food) be undiminishing and comfortable for satiating.

15.

अननं ब्रह्मा रसो बिष्णुर्भोक्ता देवो महेश्वरः ।

एवं ध्यात्वा तु यो भुङ्क्ते अन्नदोषैर्न लिप्यते ॥

Annam brahma raso visnur bhokta devo mahesvarah /
evan dhyatva tu yo bhunkte annadosair na lipyate //

One is not smeared with flaws of food if he mutters the following, Food is the Creator, taste is Vishnu and Eater is God Siva.

16.

सौवर्णं राजतं ताम्रं पात्रं शुक्तिजशङ्कजे ।

अश्मजं स्पाटिकं चैव न भेदाद् दोषमर्हति ॥

Sauvarnam rajatan tamram patram suktija-sankhaje /
asmajam sphatikan caiva na bhedad dosam arhati //

There is no fault, if a golden, silver, copper plate or a plate made of mother of pearl, conch, stone or crystal breaks (through accident).

17.

वटार्काश्वत्थपर्णेषु कुम्भीतिन्दुकपत्रयोः ।

कोविदारकरञ्जे च भुक्ता चान्द्रायणं चरेत् ॥

Vatarkasvatthaparnesu kumbhitindukapatraeyoh
kovidarakaranje ca bhuktva candrayanam caret //

One should observe the candrayana expiation, after eating on banyan, arka, pipal, kumbhi, tinduka, kovidara and karanja leaves (platter).

18.

न मुक्तकेशैर्भोक्तव्यं न नग्नः स्नानमाचरेत् ।

सुप्तव्यं नैव नग्नेन नचोच्छिष्टस्तु संविशेत् ॥

Na muktakasair bhoktavyan na nagnah snanam acaret /
suptivyan naiva nagnena na cocchistas tu samviset //

One should not dine with hair dishevelled, one should not bathe naked, one should not sleep nude, one who has eaten and not washed, should not have sexual intercourse.

19.

मौनं व्रतं महाकष्टं हुंकारेण विनश्यति ।

तथासति महादोषस्तस्मान्न नियतं चरेत् ॥

Maunam vratam mahakastam hunkarena vinasyati /
tathasati mchadosas tasman niyatan caret //

Total silence is very difficult because it is disturbed by even an inaudible 'hum' sound. If one cannot observe total silence, it should not be observed for full time (upto five morsels it should be observed).

20.

आसीनः प्राङ्मुखोऽश्नयात् वाग्यतोऽन्नमकुत्सयन् ।

अस्कन्दयंस्तन्मनाश्च भुत्का चाग्निमुपस्पृशेत् ॥

Asinah pranmukho'sniyad vagyato'nnam akutsayan /
askandayamstanmanas ca cagnim upasprset // (Baudhayana Dharmasutra ii.7.6)

Now they quote also (the following rule) He shall eat, seated with his face towards the east, silent, not despising his food, not scattering (fragments on the ground) and solely attend (to his dinner) and after he has eaten, he shall touch fire. (Buhler – SBE – p. 263)

21.

धर्मार्थकाममोक्षाणां प्राणाः संस्थितिहेतवः ।

तान्निघ्नता किन्न हतं रक्षता किन्न रक्षितम् ॥

Dharmartha-kama-moksanam pranah samsthitihetavah /
tan nighnata kin na hatam raksata kin na raksitam //

Breath is the sustaining force of religion, pecuniary gain, sexual pleasure and emancipation. What does one not destroy if he harts them (everything). What does one not preserve, if he preserves them (everything).

22.

यस्तु पाणितले भुङ्क्ते यस्तु फूत्कारसंयुतम् ।

प्रसृताङ्गुलिभिर्यश्च तस्य गोमांसवत्तु तत् ॥

Yas tu panitale bhunkte yas tu phutkarasamyutam /
prasrtangulibhir yas ca tasya gomamsavat tu tat //

He who eats from palm of hand, He who eats with labial 'phut' noise, He who eats with stretched fingers; the food for him is (sin-accruing like) beef.

23.

नाजीर्णे भोजनं कुर्यात्स्याच्च नातिबुभुक्षितः ।

हस्त्यश्वरथयानोष्ट्रप्रासादस्थो न भक्षयेत् ॥

Najirne bhojanan kuryat syac ca natibubhuksitah /
hasty-asva-ratha-yanostra-prasadastho na bhaksayet //

One should not dine when suffering from indigestion, however one should not delay to dine so that he becomes over-hungry. One should not dine while riding an elephant, horse, chariot, carriage or a camel. One should not dine while seated on a turret.

24.

श्मशानाभ्यन्तरगतो देवालयगतोऽपिवा ।

श्यनस्थो न भुंजित म पाणिस्थं न चासने ॥

Smasanabhyantaragato devalayagato'pi va /
sayanastho na bhunjita na panisthan na casane //

One should not dine inside funeral ground or temple. One should not dine (seated) on a bed, one should not dine from palm of hand, one should not dine seated on a throne or lofty seat.

25.

न सन्ध्ययोर्न मध्याहने नार्धरात्रे कदाचन ।

नार्द्रवासा नार्द्रशिरा नचायज्ञोपवीतवान् ॥

Na sandhyayor na madhyahne nardharatre kadacana /
nardravasa nardrasira na cayajnopavitavan //

(One should dine) not at morning – twilight (dawn) or at evening – twilight (dusk), not at midday or at midnight, not with wet clothes on or with head moist. One should not dine without sacred thread on.

26.

न प्रसारितपादस्तु पादारोपितपाणिमान् ।

नावसक्थिकसंस्थश्च नच पर्यङ्किकास्थितः ॥

Na prasaritapadas tu padaropitapaniman /
navasakthikasamsthas ca na ca paryankikasthitah //

(One should dine) not with stretched leg, not with palm on the thigh, not with cloth wound round the legs and not seated in a palanquin.

27.

न वेष्टितशिराश्चपि नोत्सङ्गकृतभाजनः ।

नैकवस्त्रो दुष्टमध्ये सोपानत्कः सपादुकः ॥

न चर्मोपरिसंस्थश्च चर्मरवेष्टितपार्श्ववान् ।

*Na vestitasiras ćapi notsangakrtabhajanah /
naikavastro dustamadhye sopanatkah sapadukah //
na carmoparisamsthas ca carmavestitaparsvavan /*

(One should dine) not with head-dress on, not with plate taken over thighs, nut with only dhoti on not among converted people, not with shoes or wood-wear on, not seated on hide or covering one side with hide.

28.

अननस्य जन्मकालुष्यं दुष्पक्तिं च न कुत्सयेत् ॥

ग्रासशेषं तु नाश्नीयात् पीतशेषं पिवेन्नच ।

शाकमुलपलेक्षवादि दन्तच्छेदैर्न भक्षयेत् ॥

*Annasya janmakalusyan duspaktim ca na kutsayet //
grasasesan tu nasniyat pitasesam piben na ca /
sakamulaphaleksvadi dantacchedair na bhaksyayet //*

One should not find fault with the place from which food has come (farm, dairy etc.). One should not eat the remnant from a morsel. Should not drink half-drunk water. One should not gnaw with teeth potherbs, roots, fruits, sugarcane etc.

29.

सञ्चयेन्नामन्नेन विक्षिप्तं पातूसंस्तितम् ।

बहुनामश्नतां मध्ये न चाश्नीयात् त्वरान्वितः ॥

*Sancayen nannam annena viksiptam patrasamsthitam /
bahunam asnatam madhye na casniyat tvaranvitah //*

One should not amass food served or kept in pot or plate in a heap (playing a pyramid say with laddus). One should not dine hastily among many diners (who are eating comfortably).

30.

वृथा न विकिरेदन्नं नोच्छिष्टः कुतूचिव्दूजेत् ।

न स्पृशेत् स्वशिरो विपूः सोच्छिष्टेनैव पाणिना ॥

*Vrtha na vikired annan nocchistah kutracid vrajet
na sprset svasiro viprah socchistenaiva panina //*

Brahmin should not scatter food and waste it, he should not go away without washing hands (with which he has dined). He should not touch his head with unwashed hands.

31.

तिलकल्के जलक्षीरं दधिक्षौद्रघृतानि तु ।

न त्यजेदर्धजग्धानि सक्तूंश्चाथ कदाचन ॥

Tila-kalke jala-ksiran dadhi-ksaudra-ghrtani tu /
na tyajed ardhajagdhani saktumscatha kadacana //

Half-eaten sesamum or its oil-cake, half-drunk water, milk, curds, honey and ghee, similarly baked flour should not be left over the plate.

32. (Visnu Purana iii.11.87-88)

अशनीयात्तन्मना भूतवा पूर्वं तु मधुरं रसम् ।

लवणाम्लौ तथा मध्ये कटुतिक्तादिकास्ततः ॥

प्राग्द्रवं पुरूषोऽश्नीयात् मध्ये तु कठिनाशनः ।

अन्ते पुनर्द्रवाशी च बलारोग्ये न मुञ्चति ॥

Asniyat tanmana bhutva purvan tu madhuram rasam /
lavanamlau tatha madhye katutiktadikams tatah //
Prag dravam puruso'sniyan madhye tu kathinasanah /
ante punar dravasi ca balarogye na muncati //

Let him, with an attentive mind, first taste that which has a sweet flavour, he may take salt and sour things in the middle course and finish with those which are punguent (and bitter) etc. The man who commences his meal, with fluids, then partakes of solid food and finishes with fluid again, will ever be strong and healthy. H.H. Wilson p. 247

33. (Brhaspati Smrti p.324)

आत्मार्थं भोजनं यस्य रत्यर्थं यस्य मैथनवम् ।

वृत्यर्थं यस्य चाधीतिर्निष्पलं तस्य जीवितम् ॥

Ekapanktyupevistanan duskrtam yad duratmanam /
sarvesan tat saman tavad yavat panktir na bhidyate //

Of those seated in one line for dinner, whatever sin there may be of the evil-souled, that is equally for all so long the line is not broken.

34.

हस्तं पूक्षाल्य गण्डूषं यः पिवेत्पापमोहितः ।

स दैवे चैव पित्र्ये च आत्मानं चैव सादयेत् ॥

अर्धं पीत्वा तु गण्डूपमर्धं त्याज्यं महीतले ।

रसातलगतान्नागांस्तेन प्रीणाति नित्यशः ॥

Hastam praksalya gandusam yah pibet papamohitah /
sa daive caiva pitrye ca atmanam caiva sadayet //
ardham pitva tu gandusam ardhan tyajam mahitale /
rasatalagatan nagams tena prinati nityasah //

Having washed his hands, if one drinks the entire mouthful of water carried away by sin, fails himself in honour of gods and forefathers. If one drinks half mouthful of water and sprinkles half on the ground, he always pleases the serpents in the Rasa-world.

35.

विपूस्तवेवमुपस्पृश्य पादाङ्गुष्ठे च दक्षिणे ।

हस्ताभ्यां मन्त्रवद्दद्यात् विधिवच्चावनेजनम् ॥

Vipras tvevam upasprsya padangusthe ca daksine /
hastabhyam mantravad dadyad vidhivac cavanajanam //

Having sipped water thus a Brahmin according to prescription (of religion) give water with both hands on the big toe of the right foot (of the diner).

36.

संमार्ज्यं बाहुं जानुं च गोपूदानकलं लभेत्।

भुक्त्वा नैव पूतिष्ठेत न चाप्यार्द्रेण पाणिना ॥

आचान्तोऽप्यशुचिस्तावत् यावत् पात्रमनुदधृतम् ।

उद्धृतेऽप्यशुचिस्तावत् यावन्नोन्मृज्यते मही ॥

Sammarjya bahum janum ca gopradanaphalam labhet /
bhuktva naiva pratistheta na capy ardrena panina //
Acanto'py asucis tavad yavat patram anudhrtam /
uddhrte'py asucis tavad yavan nonmrjyate mahi //

One gets the reward of giving a cow in charity it he washes his arms and knees (after eating). One should not start to go as soon as he has eaten, one should not start with wet hands.

One though he has sipped water, is impure till his plate is not lifted up. Even if this plate is lifted one is impure till the ground is not smeared (with cowdung).

37.

सुपूगं च सुपत्रं च चूर्णेन च समन्वितम् ।
अदत्वा द्विजदेवेभ्यस्ताम्बूलं वर्जयेत् बुधः ॥

Supugam ca supatram ca curnena ca samanvitam /
adattva dvijadevebhyas tambulam varjayed budhah //

Before offering a good areca-nut, a good betel-leaf with lime to Brahmin diners and divinities, a wise person should not eat betel-leaf.

38.

एकपूगं सुखारोग्यं द्विपूगं निष्फलं भवेत् ।
अतिश्रेष्ठं त्रिपूगं च ह्यधिकं नैव दुष्यति ॥

Exapugam sukharogyan dvipugan nisphalam bhavet /
atisresthan tripugam ca hy adhikan naiva dusyati //

Offering one areca-nut brings happiness and health, two areca-nuts are useless, offering three areca-nuts is very good. Even if more than three are offered it is not harmful.

39.

पर्णमूले भवेव्द्याधिः पर्णाग्रे पापसंभवः ।
चूर्णपर्णं हरेदायुः शिरा बुद्धिविनाशिनी ॥

Parnamule bhaved vyadhih parnagre papasambhavah /
curnaparnam hared ayuh sira buddhivinasini //

The lowest tip of a betel leaf causes disease. The uppermost causes sin, a broken or torn betel-leaf lessens life, the veins destroy intellect.

40.

तस्मादग्रं च मूलं च शिरा चैव विशेषतः ।
चूर्णपर्णं वर्जयित्वा ताम्बूलं खादयेत् बुधः ॥

Tasmad agram ca mulam ca siram caiva visesatah /
curnaparnam varjayitva tambulam khadayed budhah //

So, a wise person should feed betel-leaf excluding the uppermost and lowest tips, especially veins, and torn betel-leaf.

41. (Manu Smrti 4.254)

यादृशोऽस्य भवेदात्मा यादृशं च चिकिर्षितम् ।
यथा चोपचरेदेनं तथाऽऽत्मानं निवेदयेत् ॥

Yadrso'sya bhaved atma yadrsam ca cikirsitam /
yatha copecared enan tathatmanan nivedayet //

As his character is, as the work is which he desires to perform, and as the manner is in which he means to serve, even so (a voluntary slave) must offer himself. (Buhler)

42.

अवधूतमविज्ञातं सरोषं विस्मयान्विम् ।
गुरोरपि न भोक्तव्यमन्नं सत्कारवर्जितम् ॥

Avadhutam avijnatam sarosam vismayanvitam /
guror api na bhoktavyam annam satkaravarjitam //

Food served contemptuously, unacqaintedly, angrily surprisingly (oh! I did not except your presence!) and without courteousness should not be eaten, though it may be even from the preceptor.

43.

अवधूतं यदुच्छिष्टं वाग्दुष्टमपि यद्भवेत् ।

अशूद्धया हुतं दत्तमभोज्यं तद्द्विजातिभिः ॥

Avadhutam yad ucchistam vagdustam api yad bhavet /
asraddhaya hutan dattam abhojyan tad dvijatibhih //

Food served contemptuously, which is served with hand to which particles are sticking, which is found fault with spoken words, which was remnant from food part of which was offered (in sacrifice etc.). Food offered without faith should not be eaten by Brahmins.

44.

अवलि न्तस्य मूर्खस्य दुर्वृततस्य च दुर्मतेः ।

अन्नमशूद्दधानस्य यो भुङ्क्ते भ्रूणहा तथा ॥

Avaliptasya murkhasya durvrttasya ca durmateh /
annam asraddadhanasya yo bhunkte bhrunaha#tatha //

One who eats food of a proud, foolish, ill-behaved, wicked-minded or a non-believing person, is sinful like a killer of babies in embryo.

45.

अभोज्यं प्राहुराहारं शुक्तं पर्युषितं सदा ।

अन्यत्र मधुसक्तुभ्यां भक्षयेभ्यः सर्पिषो गुडात् ॥

Abhojyam prahur aharam suktam paryusitam sada /
anyatra madhu-saktubhyam bh...syebhyah sarpiso gudat //

Food excluding ready-made eatables (like laddus, sweet-meet), honey, flour of baked corn, ghee, jaggery (sugar etc.), if putrified or stale (remained overnight, hence today's morning food can be eaten till night, but yesterday-night food cannot be so), is not to be eaten.

46.

अवलीढं च मार्जारध्वाङ्क्षकुक्कुटवायसैः ।

भोजने नोपभुञ्जीत तदमेध्यं हि धर्मतः ॥

*Avalidham ca marjara-dhvanksa-kukkuta-vayasaih /
bhojane nopabhunjita tad amedhyam hi dharmatah //*

(Food) licked by cats, cranes, fowls, crows, should not be consumed while dining. It is ritualistically impure.

47.

विशुद्धमपि चाहारं दूषितं कृमिजन्तुभिः ।

केशलोमनखैर्वापि दूषितं परिवर्जयेत् ॥

*Visuddham api caharan dusitam krmi-jantubhih /
kesa-loma-nakhair vapi dusitam parivarjayet //*

Food though clean, if rendered faulty by worms and insects, or rendered blamable by hair of the head, other hair or nails is to be avoided.

48. (Manu smrti 5.2)

यज्ञार्थं ब्राह्मणैर्वध्याः प्रशस्ता मृगपक्षिणः ।

भृतयानां चैव भृत्यर्थम् अगस्त्यो ह्याचरत् पुरा ॥

वभूवुर्हि पुरोडाशा भक्षयाणां मृगपक्षिणाम् ।

पुरोणेष्वपि यज्ञेषु ब्रह्मक्षत्रसवेषु च ॥

*Yajnartham brahmanair vadhyah prasasta mrga-paksinah /
bhrtyanam caiva bhrtyartham agastyo hy acarat pura //
Babhuvur hi purodasa bhaksyanam mrga-paksinam /
puranesv api yajnesu brahmaksatrasavesu ca //*

Beasts and birds recommended (for consumption) may be slain by Brahmians for sacrifices, and in order to feed them whom they are bound to maintain, for Agestya did this of old.
For in ancient (times) the sacrificed cakes were (made of the flesh) of eatable beasts and birds at the sacrifices offered by Brahmins and Kshatriyas. (Buhler)

DICTIONARY

English	Botanical	Sanskrit	Marathi	Hindi	Gujrati	German	French
True Custard Apple of America/ Sweetsop	*Annona reticulata*	-	Ramphal	Lona	Ram-phal	Rahmaplfel	Petitcorossol
Sweet Melon or Musk Melon	*Cucumis melo*	Kalinga	Kharbuj	Khurbuj	Turbuch	Melonegurke	Cataloup
Crab-apple	*Pyrus malus*	Sebafalam	Safarchand	Seb	Sufferjang	Apfel	-
Bael fruit	*Aegle marmelos*	Bilva	Bel	Bel	Bilvaphal	-	-
Custard apple/ Sugar apple	*Annona squamosa*	Sitaphalam	Sitaphal	Sharifah	Anusa	Zue-Kerapfel	Attier
Elephant apple/ Wood apple	*Ferona elephantum*	Kapittha	Kavath	Kavat	Kotha	Elephantenatfel	Feronia geant
Pineapple	*Ananas sativus*	Annanas	Ananas	Ananas	Ananas	-	-
Jambul/ Black plum/ Blackberry	*Eugenia jambolana*	Jambu	Jambhul	Jaman/ Jam	Jambudo	Jambolinafrucht	-
Palmyra palm	*Borassus flabellifer*	Tal	Tad	Taltar	Tad	Palmfrucht	-
Sapodilla plum/ Sapta	*Achras sapota*	-	Chikku	Sapota Chikku	Chikku	Sapotafrucht	-
-	*Buchanania latifolia*	Priyal	Charoli	Piyar/ Chirenji	Charoli	-	-
Apricot	*Prunus armeniaca*	-	Jardalu	Khubani/ Jardalu		Getrocknete Aprikose	-
Banana	*Musa sapientum*	Kadali	Kela	Kela	Kela	Banane	Bananier/ Plantanier
Cashewnut	*Anacardium occidentale*	Shoephahara	Kaju	Kaju	Kaju	Katschukerne	-
Guava	*Psidium guyava*	Amrutphalam/ Bahubeeja	Peru	Amrut	Jamrukh	Guavafrucht	-
Bokhara plum/ Cherry plum	*Prunus communis*	Arook	Alubukhar	Alubokhara	Alubokhara	-	-
Raspberry	*Rubus lasiocarpus*	-	Gauriphal	-	-	Himbeere	-
Papaya	*Carica papaya*	-	Papai	Papita	Papai	Papaya/ Melonenbaum	Papayer commun
Edible date	*Phoenix dactylifera*	Pindakharjur	Khajur	Pindakhejur	Kharakia	Dattel	Palmier dattier
Fig	*Ficus carica*	Anjira	Anjir	Anjir	Anjra	Feigen	
Cluster fig Contry fig	*Ficus glomerata*	Udumbar	Udumbar	Gular	Umbaro	-	-
Grapes	*Vitis vinifera*	Draksha	Draksha	Angur	Drakshi	Edleweinrebe	Vigne-cultive
Jack fruit/ Indian jack tree	*Artocarpus integrifolia*	Panas	Phanas	Katahara	Phanas	Brotfrucht	Jaquier
Acid lime	*Citrus*	Jambeeram	Kagdi limbu	Nimbu	Limbu	Limone	-

	bergamia/ Citrus acida						
Sweet orange	*Citrus aurantium*	Swadu naring	Santra	Narengi	Narangi	Apfelsine	-
Watermelon	*Citrullus vulgaris*	Chhayaphal	Kalingad	Tarbhuz	Tarbuj	Wassermalone	Melond-eau pasteque
Citron	*Citrus medica*	Matulung	Mahalung	Maphal	Bijoura	Groblimone	
Mango	*Mangifera indica*	Amra	Amba	Am	Ambo	Mangofrucht	Manguier
Peach	*Pygeum persica/ Prunus persica*	-	-	Aru	-	Pfirsich	
Pomegranate	*Punica granatum*	Dadima	Dalimba	Anar	Dadam	Granatapfel	Grenadier cultive
Strawberry	*Frageria vesca*	-	-	-	-	Erdbeer	-
Jujube fruit	*Zizyphus jujuba*	Badari	Bor	Ber	Ber	Beere	Jujubier cotonneux
Tomato	*Lycopersicum esculentum*		Bail wangi	Bilatee baigun	Vilaiti vangan	Tomate	-
-	*Amaranthus tristis*	Mekanada	Math	Lal sag	-	-	-
-	*Amaranthus oleraceus*	Tanduliya	Tandulja	-	-	-	
Indian goosefoot/ Bathua leaves	*Chenopodium album*	Vastuk	Chakwat	Chandan betu	-	-	-
Bengal gram/ Chick pea	*Cicer arietinum*	Chanak	Harbhara	Chana	Chana	Kichererbsen	Poischi
Cow gram/ Cow pea	*Dolichos catiang*	Rajmash	Chavali	Lota	Chola	-	Dolic catjang
Horse gram	*Dolichos biflorus*	Kulatha	Kulith	Kulti	Kulti	-	Dolic-a-deux fleurs
Pea	*Pisum sativum*	Vartul	Vatana	Mattar	Vatana	Erbsen	-
Pigeon pea/ Congo pea	*Cajanus indicus*	Adhaki/ Tuvari	Tur	Arhar dal	Tuver/ Dangri	-	-
Flat bean/ Indian bean/ Goa bean	*Dolichos lablab*	Shimbi	Vaal	Sim	Val	Goa Bohnen	Chevaux defrise bean
Field pea	*Pisum arvense*	Kalay	Kala vatana	Deshi matar	Kalawatana	Schwarze Erbsen	Poisdechamps
Kidney bean	*Phaseolus aconitifolius*	Makushitha	Mataki	Math	Math	-	-
Green gram	*Phaseolus mungo*	Mudga	Mug	Moong	Mag	Rauhhaarige Bohne	Haricot mungo
Black gram	*Phaseolus radiatus*	Mash	Udid	Urid	Arad	Strahlfruchtige Bohne	Haricot radie
Lentil	*Lens esculenta*	Masur	Masur	Masoor	Masoor	Linsen	-
Chickling vetch	*Lathyrus sativus*	Triputak	Lakh	Kesari	Lang	Safran	Masaing
Cabbage	*Brassica oleracea*	-	Kobi	Kobi	Pangoli	Kohl	-
Cauliflower	*Brassica botrytis*	-	Flower	Phulkobee	-	Blumenkohl	
Carrot	*Daucus carota*	Grunjanak	Gajar	Gajar	Gajar	Karotte	Carotte cultive

Celery	*Apium graveolens*	Ajmoda	Ova	Ajmoda	-	Sellerie	-
Coriander	*Coriandrum sativum*	Dhanyaka	Dhane	Dhania	Dhania	Koriander blatter	Coriander cultive
Curry leaves	*Murraya koenigii*	Krushnarimba	Kadhee nimba	Katnim	-	Curryblatter	-
Drumstick	*Moringa olifera*	Shigru	Shavaga	Sahinjan	Sekto	-	Moringa a grainestripteres
Fenugreek	*Trigonella foenum graeceum*	Methika	Methi	Methi	Methi	-	-
Watercress	*Lepidium sativum*	Chandrashoor	Ahaliv	Chansaur	Asaliya	-	-
Indian sorrel	*Oxalis corniculata*	Changeri	Ambuti	Amrul			Oseille a trois feuilles ou du bois
-	*Agati grandiflora*	Agastya	Hadga	Hadaga	Agathiyo	-	-
Lettuce	*Lactuca scariola*		Kahu	Salad	Kahu	Kopfsalat	Laitue cultivec
Mint	*Mentha arvenis*	Putiha	Pudina	Pudina	Pudina	Minze	-
Dill leaves	*Peucedanum graveolens*	Mishreya	Shepu	Sowa	Surva-nu-bi	Gartendill Dillblatter	Persil des marais
Red sorrel	*Hibiscus sabdariffa*	-	Lal-ambadi	Patwa	Lal ambadi	Rothe sabderiffe	Ketmie Acide/ Osille rough de Guince
Spinach	*Spinacia oleracea*	Palakya	Palak	Palak	Palak	Spinat	Epinard Cornu
Malabar night shade	*Basella alba*	Potaki	Velbondi	Poi	Maya-ki-baji	-	-
Common asparagus	*Asparagus officinalis*	Shatavari	Shatavari	Marchuba	-	Asparagus	-
Spreading hog weed	*Boe-rhaavia diffusa*	Punarnava	Ghetuli	Thikri	Vakha-khapar	-	-
Sweet Basil	*Ocimum basilicum*	Visha tulsi	Sabja Tulsi	Sabzah	-	Basilienkraut	Basilic cultive
Indian gooseberry	*Emblica officinalis*	Amalaki	Avla	Aoula	Amla	-	Phyllanthe Emblic
White pumpkin/ White gourd melon	*Benincasa hispida/ Benincasa cerifera*	Kushmanda	Kohala	Golkaddu	Kohala	-	-
Bitter gourd	*Momordica charantia*	Sushavi	Karla	Karela	Karela	Bittergurke	Momordique charantia
Bitter bottle gourd	*Lagenaria vulgaris*	Katutumbi	Kadubhopla	Lauki	Dudhi	Kurbis	Gourde
Brinjal,/ Eggplant	*Solanum melongena*	Vartak	Vangi	Begun	Baigan	Eierfruchte Auhergine	-
Broad bean	*Faba vulgaris*	-	Kale vaal	Seo-chana Bakla	-	Schwarze Bohnen	-
Double bean/ Lima pole bean	*Phaseolus lunatus*	-	Double bee	-	-	Doppelbohnen	-

Common cucumber	*Cucumis sativus*	Trapusha	Kakdi	Khira	Kakri	Gurke	-
Red gourd/ Spanish gourd/ Great pumpkin	*Cucurbita maxima*	Punyalatha/ Dadhiphala	Lal bhopla	Pila kohola/ Mitha kaddu	Pilun-kohalun	Kurbis	Gourge
Patol/ Wash sponge/ Smooth luffa	*Luffa aegyptiaca*	Raj-koshataki	Ghosali	Ghiaturai	Turia	-	-
Cluster bean/ Field vetch	*Cyamopsis psoralioides*	Gorani	Gawar	Gowar	Guar	-	-
Common French bean	*Phaseolus vulgaris*	-	Shravan ghevda	Bakla/ Sem	-	Bohnen	Petitefeve
Okra/ Edible hibiscus/ Ladies finger	*Abelmoschus esculentus*	Tindisha	Bhendi	Bhindi	Bhinda	Okra	-
Ridge gourd	*Luffa acutangula*	Koshataki	Dodka	Torai/ Jinga	Sirola Turiya	Scarfeckige gurke	-
Snake gourd	*Trichosanthes anguina*	Chinchida	Padval	Chichoda	Pandola	Schlangenkurbiss	
Wild snake gourd	*Trichosanthes dioica*	Patol	Kadu padwal	Parwar		-	Trichosanthes conturne
Soya bean	*Glycine soja*			Bhatwan	-	Sojabohnen	-
Sword bean/ Jack bean	*Canavalia ensiformis*	Mahashimbi	Pathave	Kadasambal	Abao	Schwertbohnen	
Turnip	*Brassica campestris*	Raktasarshap	Shiras/ Shalgham	Shulgum	-	Rube/ WeiBrube	-
Bell pepper/ Spanish pepper/ Monstrous pepper	*Capsicum grossum*	-	Bhopla mirchi	-			-
Beetroot/ Sugar beet	*Beta vulgaris*	-	Beet	Chukander	-	Rotrube	-
Colocasia	*Colocasia antiquorum*	-	Arvi	Arvi	-	Schild formiger	Colocasie de L Inde
Potato	*Solanum tuberosum*		Batata	Alu	Papeta	Kartoffel	Pomme de terre
Onion	*Allium cepa*	Palandu	Kanda	Piyaz	Dungri kando	Zwiebel	-
Radish	*Raphanus sativus*	Moolaka	Mula	Mula	Muri	Rettich	Raifort cultive
Sweet potato	*Ipomoea batatas*	Raktalu	Ratali	Sakharkand	Sakaria	SuBkartoffel	Truffle douce/ Potate de Maluga
Yam	*Dioscorea bulbifera*	Suran	Suran	Zaminkand	Goradu	Rubenkohl	
Almond	*Prunus amygdalus*	Vatam	Badam	Badam	Badam	Mandelkerne	
Coconut	*Cocos nucifera*	Narikel	Naral	Nariyal	Naliar	Kokosnuss	Cocotier
Indian water Chestnut/ Indian caltrop	*Trapa bispinosa*	Shrungatak	Shingada	Singhara	Singari	Wasserkastanie	Noix aquatique Corniole
Indian walnut	*Aleurites*	Akshota	Ramakrod	Akhrot	-	Walnuss	-

	moluccana						
Pistachionut	*Pistacia vera*	-	Pista	Pista	-	Pistaziennuss	-
Groundnut/ Peanut	*Arachis hypogaea*	Bhuchanak	Bhuimug	Mungphali	Bhoising	Erdnuss	-
Walnut	*Juglans regia*	Akshota	Akrod	Akhroot	-	Wallnuss	Noyer cultive Gognier
Sunflower	*Helianthus annuus*	Suryamukhi/ Adityabhakta	Suryaphul	Surajmukhi	Surajmukh	Sonnenblumenkerne	-
Castrol oil plant	*Ricinus communis*	Erand	Erand	Endi	Diveli	Rizinussamen	Ricin
Cotton	*Gossypium herbaceum*	Karpas	Kapus	Kapas	-	Baumwollsamen	Cotonnier Herbace
Sesame	*Sesamum indicum*	Til	Til	Til	Tal	Sesamsamen	Sesame
Olive	*Olea europaea*	-	-	-	-	Olivenol	-
Safflower	*Carthamus tinctorius*	Kusumba	Kardi	Kusum	Kusumbi	-	Cartheme Faux safran
Bajra spiked millet	*Pennisetum typhoideum*	Varjari	Bajri	Bajra	Bajri Sejji		
Linseed/ Flax tree	*Linum usitatissimum*	Uma	Javas	Tisi/ Alsi	Alshi	Flachs	Lincuttive
Barley	*Hordeum vulgare*	Yav	Jav/ Satu	Jave/ Jan	Cheno	Gerste	Orge anguleuse
Oat	*Avena sativa*	-	Jai	-	-	Hafer	
Rice	*Oryza sativa*	Tandula	Tandul	Dhan Chaval	Chokha	Reis	
Jowar	*Sorghum vulgare*	-	Jwari	Jawar	-	Hirse	-
Wheat	*Triticum sativum*	Godhuma	Gahu	Gehun	Gehu	Weizen	-
Maize/ Indian corn	*Zea mays*	Yavanal	Maka	Makka/ Bhutta	Makai	Mais korner	-
Small millet/ Broomcorn millet	*Fanicum milliaceum*	China	Dhengali/ vari	China	Gadio	Achte Hirse	Millet round
Italian millet	*Setaria italica*	Kangu	Kang, Rala	Kangu	Kang	Italienische Hirse	
Indian millet/ Korakan	*Eleusine coracana*	Soma	Nachani	Makra	Bavto/ Navto		-
Rough chaff tree/ Prickly chaff flower	*Achyranthes aspera*	Apamarga	Aghada	Latjira/ Chirchira	Safed aghed	-	-
Asafoetida	*Ferula foetida*	Hingu	Hing	Hingra	Hing	Asafotedea	Ferule asafoetida
Cardamom	*Elettaria cardamomum*	Ela	Veldoda	Chhoti elachi	Elachi	Kardomon	-
Chillies	*Capsicum aunum*	Lanka	Lavangi mirchi	Jhal	Marchi	Pepperoni	-
Cinnamon	*Cinnamomum zeylanicum*	Twak	Dalchini	Dalchini	Dalchini	Zimt	Cannelle
Clove	*Eugenia caryophyllata*	Devakusum	Lavang	Laung	Lavang	Znelke	Girofla
Nutmeg	*Myristica fragrans*	Jatiphal	Jayaphal	Jayphal	Jayiphal	Muscatnuss	Muscadier/ Musque
Cumin seed	*Cuminum cyminum*	Jeerak	Jeera	Safed jeera	Safed jiraun	Kummel	Anisacre/ Cumin

							officinal
Garlic	*Allium sativum*	Rason	Lasun	Lasan	Lasan	Knoblauch	-
Ginger	*Zingiber officinale*	Shunthi	Sunth	Sonth	Adu	Ingwer	Gingembre
Bishops weed	*Carum roxburghianum*	Ajmoda	Ova	Ajowan	Ajamo	Indisches Falenohr	-
Black pepper	*Piper nigrum*	Marich	Mire	Kalimirich	Kalomirich	Pfeffer	Poivre
Indian sweet fennel Fennel	*Foeniculum vulgare*	Madhurika	Badishep	Badi saunf	Warialli	Fenchel	-
White mustard	*Brassica alba*	Shweta sarshap	Pandhari mohari	Safedrai	Safed rai	Weisser senf	Moutar de Clanche
Brown mustard	*Brassica juncea*	Rajika	Mohri	Rai	Rai	Senfkorner	-
Black mustard	*Brassica nigra*	Sarshap	Mohori	Kolorai Makra rai	Rai	Schwarze senfkorner	Moutarde Noire
Tamarind	*Tamarindus indica*	Tintidik	Chinch	Imbli	Amli	Tamarind	Tamarinier
Cassia clmmamon	*Cinnamomum tamala*	Tejapatra	Tamalpatra	Tejpat	-	-	-
Turmeric	*Curcuma longa*	Haridra	Halad	Haldi	Halder	Gelbgewurz Kurkuma	Curcuma long
Arecanut	*Areca catechu*	Pooga	Supari	Supari	Supari	Arekanuss	Noix d'Arec
Betel leaf pepper	*Piper betle*	Nagavalli	Nagvel	Pan Tamboli	Pan	Betelblatt	Betel
Sago	*Sagus leaves*	-	Sabudana	Sabudana	-	Sagokorner	-
Sugarcane	*Saccharum officinarum*	Ikshu	Oos	Ganna	Sherdi	Zuckerrohr	Kanne a Sucre
Honey	*Apis mellifica*	Madhu	Madh	Madha Shahad	Madha	Honig	-
Yeast	*Cervisi actermeutum*	-	-	Khamir	-	Hefe	-
Camphor	*Camphora officinarum*	Karpoor	Kapur	Kapur	Kapur	Kampher	camphre
Rock salt	*Sodium chloride impura*	Saindhav	Saindhav	Sendhalon	sindhaluna	Natri chloricum	-

BOOKS AND THESES

Books

1. Ayurveda Aahar, Prof. Dr. P. H. Kulkarni

The book elaborates the principles of Ayurveda, digestion rules of consumption of food, properties of food material etc. It has classic deascription about the effects of food on mind. The book has separate chapters on milk and water. Dietary regimen has been described for various diseases.

2. Ayurvedic Indian Cooking, Dr Sunanda Ranade

The book has been divided in three parts. In first part, basic principles of Ayurveda especcially with relation to food effects have been explained. In second part, Ayurvedic concepts of nutrition, roles and regulations of eating, contradictory food etc. have been mentioned. In part three, various recipes, beverages, snacks, leafy vegetables, rice, chapati, sweets, etc. and its effects on doshas have been explained. Over all 100 recipes have been explained in the book.

3. The Ayurvedic Cook Book, Amadea Morningstar with Urmila Desai

The book gives a fresh new perspective on this ancient art of self-healing. Over 250 tastes - tested recipes are specifically designed to balance each constitution, with an emphasis on simplicity, ease and sound nutrition. Recipes range from exotic Indian meals to old American favourites. It includes an in depth discussion of Ayurvedic nutrition, tridoshic perspective and way to make dietary changes that last. It is a personalised guide to good nutrition and health. The book is divided into three parts with general information such as basic principles, diet etc. Then follow the recipes and appendices.

4. The Healing Diet, Victor Horbest and Beverly Jacobson

The book explains how to reduce your risks and live a longer and healthier life if you have a family history of cancer, heart disease, hypertension, diabetes, alcoholism, obesity, food allergies etc. It gives you all the information you need to create a nutritional program tailored to your personal needs.
In an easy to follow style, it tells you;

a. How to create a family medical tree
b. How to use the information to create a diet tailored to your personal need.
c. Included are specific guidelines and nutrition pathways and chronic diseases.

Hence the book tells the secret of right eating, good feeling and longer life.

5. Fruits and Vegetables in Ancient India, Dr. P. V. Sharma

The book has given a detail summary of different fruits and vegetables. The introduction does explain the historic background of food mentioned in all the ancient texts. The first chapter consists of 84 different fruits, followed with dietary preparation from fruit, liquid preparations from food, fermented beverages, fruits used as mouth refreshing agents. The second chapter explains 271 vegetables. The entire book is a classical collection of references of food material.

6. Aahar aani Madhumeha (Food & diabetes), In Marathi by Dr. K.V. Panse

The book has information and definition regarding diabetes, history, signs and symptoms: quality and quantity wise description of diet in diabetes, information regarding exercise, medicines, etc. The author has described in terms of modern medicine.

7. Taak va aarogya (Buttermilk and health), In Marathi by Vd. Ganesh Pandurangshastri Paranjpe

Author has explained the benefits of buttermilk on health. He has given the method of preparation, contraindications, medicinal values of buttermilk, quantity of buttermilk according to age.

8. Aahar (Diet), In Hindi by Kaviraj Laxminarayan Sharma

Author has elaborately explained the theory of proteins, carbohydrates, fats, minerals etc. he has furnished a detailed information regarding milks and milk products of cow and buffallo, fruits, vegetables, tea, coffee, fish, eggs, meats etc.

9. Khadya ki nayee vidhi (Food recipes of the modern world), In Hindi by Kularanjan Mukherjee

Beverages including alcohol, dietetic regimen according to the disease, spices and disease, diet according to age, fruits and health, dietetic regimen in pregnancy, dietetic elements such as carbohydrates, proteins, fats, etc. are explained in detail.

10. Aahar our swasthya (Diet for health), In Hindi by Dr. Hiralal N.D.

The book is divided into 3 volumes. The book has description about the human physiology, dietetic elements such as proteins, fats, carbohydrates etc., quantity of food and dietetic regimen according to seasons.

11. Aarogya Aani Aahar (Health and Diet), In Marathi by Prof. Shanta Kelkar

The book has detailed description about diet according to age. The author has classified the food items into various groups such as fruits, roots and tubers, milk, spices etc. The book also contains a description regarding the elements of diet.

12. Handbook of food and Nutrition, Dr. M. Swaminathan

The author has given a detailed description of the following subjécts-
Nutrition of Pre-School children, Nutrition of Industrial workers, geriatric nutrition, diet in obesity, processed supplementary food and novel foods, effect of cooking and heat processing on the nutrition value of food etc. Alongwith this description, he has also given information regarding the essential nutrients.

13. Child Nutrition- Problems and Prospects, Vol I & II, M. Varma, B. Mathur, A. Goyle, M. Agrawal, G. Singh.

The authors have elaborately explained nutritional status, health profile of rural and urban children. This whole is sponsored by UNICEF.

14. Food and Nutrition: Facts and Figures (English), Dr. L. C. Gupta, Dr.(Mrs) Kusum Gupta & Abhisek Gupta

Common person is the aim of this book. The author has classified the food in proteins, carbohydrates, fats etc. Malnutrition, toxins of food (Lythyrism, afla toxicosis etc.), food adulteration etc. and special diets in specific diseases are explained here.

15. Kha Pya, Bare Wha (Marathi) (Eat & Live better), Prof. Dr. P. H. Kulkarni

The author has explained dietary regimen for almost all the commonly found disorders. He has also described a specific diet pattern for healthy long life.

List of other Books

- Chemistry of food and nutrition by sherman HC, McMillan Co. New York
- Biochemistry and physiology of nutrition vol: 1&2, edited by Bourne GH & Kidder GW, Academic press. Inc. New York.
- Nutrition in health and disease by cooper LF, Barer EM, Mitchell HS, Rynbergen HJ, JB Lippincot Co. Philadelphia & Montreal.
- Handbook of nutrition - A Symposium prepared under the auspices of the council on foods & nutrition of the American medical Association. The Blackiston Co. Inc. New York, Toronto.
- Nutrition and physical fitness by Boert LJ, WB Saunders Co. Philadelphia & London.
- Food the yearbook of agriculture 1959, US Department of Agriculture Washington D.C.
- Nutrition by Chaney - Publisher Mifflin Co. Boston.
- Feeding the family by Rose MS, McMillon Co. New York.
- Nutrition in India, VN Patwardhan - Indian Journal of Medical Sciences. Mumbai 4.
- Balanced diet and nutritive value of common recipes - central food technological research Inst. Mysore.
- Elements of food biochemistry by Peterson, Skinner & Strong, Prentice Hall Inc. New York.

Thesis

1. A special study of the functions of pachakagni with special reference to the difference in opinions of charaka and sushruta samhita.
   M.D. Ayu.Vachaspati
   Vd. Mandar Laxman Bedekar

In hypothesis the Research scholar projects that the scholars of Dhanvantari school of thought might have observed the functions of the pachakagni in operated individuals. In discussion concept of Agni, its' physiological assistance i.e., Pittadhara - Kala - Grahani - Saman Vayu has been discussed.

The sacrifice of the 'dravata' by the pachakagni, fluid and electrolyte balance, primarily water retention, early sodium retention, late sodium retention, post operative nausea and vomiting etc. are explained in detail. Considering the limitations the research scholar has made a brief conclusion with the hypothesis highlighting the scope of the topic. research scholar suggests that it will help the scientist to frame the do's and don'ts for the patients who are likely to undergo a surgical procedure. It proves that the pachakagni is considered to be responsible for the maintenance of health. It will help in deciding the amount of food for a particular individual.

2. Kostha Parikshan and Dosha Prakriti Sambandha ek Abhyasa
   Vd. Meenakshi Ashok Khandar

Out of 100 patients observed 85% cases have been found of utkat dosha in kostha and prakriti. In 15% cases similarity in kosth parikshana done by purish mala parikshana and kostha parikshana, confirmed by virechana.
Conclusion of utkata dosha in prakriti can be done by kostha parikshan and purish. Koshtha parikshana is confirmed by virechana, but it can not be confirmed 100%, if virechan vidhi is done with purvakarma (snehan and swedan). It will be more confirmative kostha and will be helpful to ascertain utkat dosha in prakriti.

References

Harisastri Paradakara(Ed.) 1982 (originally Published in 1939) collatee by Late Dr. Anna Moreswara Kunte & Krsna Ramchandra Sastri Navare *Astangahrdayam Composed by Vagabhata*, Chaukhambha Orientalia, Varanasi.

Ibhavaprakash Nighantu

Yadavji Trikamji Acharya (Ed.) 1981 (originally published in 1941) *The Charak Samhita of Agnivesa Revised by Charaka & Dridhabala with the Ayurveda – Dipika Commentary of Chakrapanidatta*, Munsiram Monoharlal Publishers Pvt. Ltd., New Delhi

Yadavji Trikamji Acharya (Ed.) *Susruta Samhita of Susruta with the Nibandhasangraha Commentary of Sri Dalhanacharya*, Chaukhambha Orientalia, Varanasi

K.M. Nadkarni (Revised and Enlarged by Mr. A.K. Nadkarni) *Indian Materia Medica (Vol I & Vol. II)*, Dhootpapeshwar Prakashan Ltd., Panvel.

P.H. Kulkarni 1996 *Ayurveda Aahar/ Diet*, Ayurveda Education Series, Pune

Vishnu Mahadev Gogte 1982 *Dravyaguna Vidnyan (Ayurvedik Materia Medica)*, Continental Prakashan, Pune